Caregiving in Alzheimer's and Other Dementias

Caregiving in Alzheimer's and Other Dementias

Eric Pfeiffer, M.D.

FOREWORD BY
Gayle Sierens

Yale UNIVERSITY PRESS

New Haven & London

The information and suggestions contained in this book are not intended to replace the services of your physician or caregiver. Because each person and each medical situation is unique, you should consult your own physician to get answers to your personal questions, to evaluate any symptoms you may have, or to receive suggestions for appropriate medications.

The author has attempted to make this book as accurate and up to date as possible, but it may nevertheless contain errors, omissions, or material that is out of date at the time you read it. Neither the author nor the publisher has any legal responsibility or liability for errors, omissions, out-of-date material, or the reader's application of the medical information or advice contained in this book.

Yale University Press books may be purchased in quantity for educational, business, or promotional use. For information, please e-mail sales.press@yale.edu (U.S. office) or sales@yaleup.co.uk (U.K. office).

Designed by James J. Johnson.
Set in Swift type by Integrated Publishing Solutions.
Printed in the United States of America.

Library of Congress Cataloging-in-Publication Data
Pfeiffer, Eric, 1935–
   Caregiving in alzheimer's and other dementias / Eric Pfeiffer, M.D. ; foreword by Gayle Sierens, News Anchor, NBC-TV, Tampa, Florida.
      pages cm
   Includes index.
   ISBN 978-0-300-20798-9 (pbk. : alk. paper) 1. Alzheimer's disease–Patients–Care. 2. Caregivers. I. Title.
   RC523.P436 2015
   616.8'31–dc23   2014033323

A catalogue record for this book is available from the British Library.

This paper meets the requirements of ANSI/NISO Z39.48–1992 (Permanence of Paper).

10 9 8 7 6 5 4 3 2 1

Contents

Part II. Learning about Your Loved One's Condition

Part III. Providing Care for Your Loved One

Part IV. Taking Care of Yourself

Foreword

Nearly thirty years ago I had the distinct pleasure of meeting Dr. Eric Pfeiffer. As a television news reporter and anchor, it was my job to share with our viewers the latest breakthroughs in medicine. Here in Florida, a great deal of that news deals with our aging population, of which I am now a part. I had the good fortune to meet and interview this brilliant man whose passion it is to better the lives of the elderly, and help the rest of us understand what they are facing and in many cases, already dealing with. Little did I know that I would be one of those people.

I am the only child of a mother who has now moved through all the stages of Alzheimer's. It's hard to understand that world unless you are in the middle of it. But Dr. Pfeiffer has given us not only a glimpse into that world with his book *Caregiving in Alzheimer's and Other Dementias;* he has taken us by the hand and given us a step-by-step guide for how to walk that path. He has equipped us with courage and armed us with information. I am grateful that this most useful tool is now available as other caregivers make their way through such a puzzling disease. I am thankful as well for the fact that Dr. Pfeiffer continues his compassionate efforts on behalf of those who have the disease, and those who care for their loved ones.

On April 6, 2014, my mother breathed her last breath, as my daughter and I hovered over her hospital bed. It had been a four-day vigil (actually, a ten year and four-day vigil) that ended with both tears and relief. I have a sense of relief that she is no longer trapped in a body that still worked in many ways, but a mind that didn't. I do say that every single day I miss her sweet smile and the tight grip she was still able to muster around my hand each day. Now instead of a schedule that revolved around being by her side every day, I find a void. I can fill the time easily with my crazy, busy life, just not the caregiving experience that made me feel so needed. As Dr. Pfeiffer so eloquently describes in his final chapter of this book, entitled "Recovery from Caregiving," I did indeed learn how strong and resourceful I can be. Alzheimer's taught me many things. Mostly it taught me we must find a cure. Recovering and redefining my worth is now my work in progress, after more than a decade of planning every day around my mother's disease.

—Gayle Sierens, News Anchor,
NBC-TV, Channel 8, Tampa, Florida

Introduction

I F YOU are a caregiver of someone with Alzheimer's disease or another form of dementia, or if you are considering becoming a caregiver of someone afflicted with Alzheimer's disease, this book is for you. It is intended as your personal guide to a journey the likes of which you have never before experienced. Even if you have raised children, taught school, supervised employees, or have in other ways taken on responsibility for someone else, becoming an Alzheimer's caregiver will challenge you in ways you could never have imagined. If you have never been charged with caring for someone else, you will find that caring for someone with Alzheimer's disease creates demands and opportunities of an entirely different order than anything else you have ever encountered—simply because Alzheimer's is a disease like no other. Its manifestations will change continually and progressively before your very eyes, and before you know it, you too will be changed forever by having been a caregiver to someone with this disease. You may even be changed for the better, in ways that I will explain throughout the book.

The reason I have written this book is that I have seen this disease at close range in my role as the treating physician for thousands of Alzheimer's patients. In that role I have also had the opportunity of seeing thousands of caregivers deal with the challenges presented by this disease, and have learned from them a great deal about caregiving. In particular, I have seen caregivers develop and share innovative approaches, creative attitudes, and ingenious techniques that allowed them to discover strengths they never knew they possessed and bring those to their important job of helping their loved ones. Many of them have truly become modern-day heroes, as they learned, through trial and error, and from each other, what worked and what didn't work. It is their cumulative wisdom and experience that I employ to light your way as you embark on the remarkable journey that lies ahead.

In this book I will also convey to you some of the

fundamental knowledge we have today about Alzheimer's disease. It is a disease of the brain, not simply a manifestation of aging. To date we do not fully understand the causes of this remarkable disease, but real progress is being made toward our goal of stopping and maybe someday even reversing its devastating effects. Understanding the nature of this disease will help you as you assume your role as a caregiver for someone with Alzheimer's. And it will help you to make a positive difference in the life of your loved one.

This book began as a much slimmer volume entitled *The Art of Caregiving in Alzheimer's Disease*. It was first published by Lulu Press in 2011, and later appeared as both a print book and also as an e-book on Amazon.com. Many caregivers and caregiver groups relied on its advice (some even described it as a "lifeline"), and it was well reviewed, but it did not attain the widespread distribution I had hoped for given the millions of caregivers involved in dementia care. Therefore I was extremely grateful when Jean Thomson Black at Yale University Press accepted this book for publication in a much expanded form, with the aim of reaching the much wider audience the topic deserves. As an experienced publisher in the arena of health and wellness, Yale University Press is in a unique situation to deliver on this promise.

Although the main focus of this book is Alzheimer's disease, other forms of dementia will be dealt with as well. I will point out how these other dementias differ from Alzheimer's disease, but please be advised that whenever I use the term Alzheimer's disease, much of what is presented applies to other forms of dementia too. (It would be awkward to write "Alzheimer's disease and other dementias" over and over again.) Indeed, while this book deals specifically with caregiving in dementing disorders, many of the principles presented here also apply to caregiving for virtually all chronic diseases and disabilities.

Thank you for opening this book and for opening your mind to the suggestions and guidance offered here. The insights provided are intended not only to help you become a skilled, knowledgeable caregiver to your loved one, but also to nurture you as a person during this challenging period of life. If you are reading this as a caregiver struggling with a new diagnosis or a sudden decline in your loved one's abilities, don't panic. This book will point you to resources that can help you and your loved one now and through the months and years ahead.

PART I

Understanding the Caregiver Role

Chapter 1

What Is a Caregiver?

A CAREGIVER does those things that a sick or disabled person can no longer do independently. In other words, what a caregiver does depends on what that other person needs to have done for him or her, which in turn will depend on the stage or severity of the illness or disability. In some cases, and at some stages of a disease, caregiving may involve only a little bit of help: steadying the person's gait, combing his or her hair, helping with getting dressed or making it to the bathroom on time. In other cases it can be much more involved and labor-intensive, to the point where the caregiver does virtually everything for the other person.

Why Become a Caregiver?

The only reason you would consider becoming a caregiver is that someone near and dear to you needs care and you are the only logical person to provide that care. Why? Because you love that person or are committed to that person in some profound way, most commonly through blood or marriage. Consider what taking on the job of caregiver would mean to you. Don't you have your own life to live? Wouldn't giving up a good part of your own life to take care of another person full-time be asking rather a lot? Indeed it is. So why would you want to become a caregiver?

Nobody Wants to Be a Caregiver

In truth, nobody *wants* to be a caregiver. The fact that someone dear to you is in need of such care is a painful one to face. You will become a caregiver only because the role is thrust upon you by fate or circumstances, or because of who you are and what is possible for you at this time of your life. So how and why is it that you are even considering this exhausting and often underappreciated job?

There is no law that says you have to be the one who becomes the patient's caregiver. You can decide that it is simply not something you can or want to do, and then someone else will have to take on this task: another relative, a friend, or even a paid care manager. Usually this choice will have to be faced fairly early on in the course of the patient's disease. The fact that you are reading this book seems to indicate that you are seriously leaning in the direction of taking on this role. But remember, it is a choice. You can still change your mind before it is too late.

For my part, I am going to try to do everything possible to help you carry out this choice with skill and elegance, yes, even with joy.

Caregivers Are a Lifeline to Their Patients

Without caregivers, patients with Alzheimer's disease could not find their way to the doctor. They could not accurately provide their own history, neither their medical history nor the history of their lives. And they could not convey the extent of their memory problems nor the behavioral problems that accompany their memory deficits. What caregivers do is vitally important to the patient. Their duties may include preparing meals and giving the patient medications on the prescribed schedule. Above all, they provide emotional support as well as love and affection to the patient. Caregivers also help patients to make decisions or, later in the disease when the patient can no longer participate in decision-making, make decisions on the patient's behalf. Caregivers serve as advocates for the patient, too. They become the guardian angel to the patient, hovering nearby and keeping the patient from missteps or harm. But caregivers should take over only what their patients can no longer do independently, and encourage patients to exercise all the skills they still possess.

Caregivers and Doctors: An Essential Partnership

Caregivers, almost as much as physicians, are decision-makers concerning when patients begin and whether they continue treatment. For this reason it is critical that caregivers understand the nature of the illness as well as the benefits, limitations, and potential side effects of all available treatments. (I will discuss what the currently available treatments can and cannot accomplish in Chapter 9.)

After treatment begins, caregivers must also work with doctors to observe and report beneficial or adverse changes in the patient's response. This is critical since patients may have widely varying reactions to medications. Caregivers are the ones to refill or renew the patient's prescriptions and carry out any other instructions given by the prescribing doctor. Since Alzheimer's disease can last anywhere from two to twenty-five years, doctors and caregivers need to establish a long-term partnership of mutual trust and respect. For this reason I advise that at each visit the doctor and caregiver spend some time with each other away from the patient, so that they both can feel free to raise any issues that would be uncomfortable to discuss in the patient's presence.

Caregivers Assure Patients' Quality of Life

While doctors can diagnose and make treatment recommendations, the day-to-day quality of life rests largely in the hands of the caregiver. Caregivers' efforts to provide continuity, dignity, pleasure, social interaction, a stable environment, and freedom from unwanted surprises make a huge difference in the life of an Alzheimer's patient. In fact, what the caregiver does determines in large part how patients deal with their fate: either calm acceptance of the disease or some form of lashing out against the caregiver and the rest of the world.

Some people are natural-born caregivers. They do all the right things, without instruction. But other caregivers don't know where to start, and may need a lot of help. I am hoping that this book will provide some of the necessary guidance. I want to convey all that I know about the illness, about available treatments, and how to manage disruptive behaviors when they occur. I also want to make you aware that patients with any form of dementia may undergo significant personality changes as part of the illness, changes that will require that caregivers adapt.

At the University of South Florida we have developed a series of caregiver classes to teach family members about the illness, about available treatments and techniques for managing disruptive behaviors, and about available community resources such as daycare and respite care. These classes also teach how to prepare legally and financially for the caregiver experience, with information about durable power of attorney, health surrogate instruments, and living wills. In our caregiver classes we use the natural-born caregivers as teachers and models of care provision. To find caregiver classes in your community, check with your local chapter of the Alzheimer's Association. If no such caregiver classes exist, you might ask your doctor or your memory disorder clinic to start them; participants in our caregiver classes have called them true lifesavers.

Some Caregivers Risk Becoming Patients Themselves

Given the demands and stresses of caregiving, it should not be surprising that some caregivers may become patients themselves, at times succumbing to depression, burnout (sometimes called compassion fatigue), or self-neglect. To minimize the risk of this happening, caregivers need emotional support, recognition, encouragement, suggestions for coping techniques, and information about their role as caregivers. This is an issue of such great importance that I have devoted an entire part of this book to it (see Chapters 17 through 20). But right up front there are a few things that caregivers need to understand and do even before they are involved in the thick of caregiving:

- You, the caregiver, must take responsibility for maintaining your own health, mental health, and sense of well-being. Should you fail to do so, you will not be able to provide the care that is needed. Instead your patient will decline more rapidly and possibly require premature admission to a healthcare facility, at great financial and emotional cost.
- You need to avail yourself of all the help that may be available to you. This includes joining a caregiver support group in the earliest stages of caregiving, as well as asking for and accepting practical and emotional support from other family members and from your friends.
- Keep your patient's doctor apprised of how you yourself are doing, and ask his or her advice for keeping you feeling and functioning well.

The Stages of Caregiving

Just as there are distinct stages of Alzheimer's disease, described in detail in Chapters 13 through 15, there are also distinct stages of caregiving.

Stage 1: Coping with the Diagnosis

Being told that your spouse, mother, father, or someone else near and dear to you has Alzheimer's disease can be a shocking experience. Most people have some idea, accurate or not, of what this diagnosis implies. And none of it is good. Immediately, there are a lot of questions to be answered: What is Alzheimer's disease? How severe is the disease at this point, or at what stage is the affected person? What treatments are available and when should treatment begin? Is Alzheimer's disease inherited? Many more questions will occur to you and you should try to get every one of them answered. Some can be answered by your doctor. For others, a search on the internet is in order: try WebMD.com, for starters. Then read some books on Alzheimer's disease. In addition to the book you are now reading, read *The 36-Hour Day* by Nancy Mace and Peter Rabins, which has been described as "the bible" on Alzheimer's disease.

Stage 2: Deciding Who Will Be the Caregiver

Figuring out who will care for your loved one is a critical decision for you, for the affected person, and for anyone else considered a candidate for the caregiver role. Caregiving can be done well by other family members, very close friends, or even professional caregivers. Depending on your relationship to the patient, you will need to decide first whether you are the "logical" person to take on this role, and second, whether you are willing and able to do so. If not, you will probably need to find and designate an alternate caregiver.

Stage 3: Caregiving at Home

Caregiving in the patient's home will be the longest and most complicated period of caregiving, as the patient progresses through the various stages of the disease (early, middle, and late). The majority of this book is devoted to serve as a guidebook for this stage of caregiving, though the other stages of caregiving are also very important.

Stage 4: Considering Residential Placement

This stage of caregiving, dealing with the decision to consider residential placement of the patient, is considered in Chapter 16. It can be very difficult emotionally for the caregiver and others in the patient's support network.

Stage 5: Caregiving during Residential Placement

Once the patient has been moved into a residential facility, it may seem at first that the caregiver role has ended or is at least markedly diminished. But this is far from the case. The caregiver's role certainly changes during this transition, but it nevertheless continues in full. Now it involves visiting the patient in the residential setting at regular intervals—perhaps daily, or on another schedule, depending on distances involved and any other commitments the caregiver may have. It still is all about assuring the best care for the patient, only now any number of other people and a whole new organization are involved. Especially in the early phases of residential placement, the patient needs to be assured that you are still involved as he or she adjusts to a whole new environment and to a whole array of new people who will provide care. During this time you may be besieged by demands from the patient to be taken "home." You may also face anger and blame from the patient for having been moved to a care facility, as well as all sorts of requests from facility staff. Please remember that this is a period of transition for everyone involved. The most helpful advice for this stage of caregiving may come to you from other members of a caregiver support group who have gone through the same experience, and from the doctor who is caring for your patient. You will find more about how members of a caregiver support group can help in Chapter 18.

Stage 6: Dealing with the Death of the Patient

Eventually your patient will die. During this stage, entirely new feelings of grief, and to some extent feelings of relief, will require special attention. You can read more about this transition in Chapter 19.

Stage 7: Recovering from Caregiving

Recovering from the exhausting role of being a caregiver to a patient with Alzheimer's disease or another dementia involves its own challenges. The transition is so important that I have devoted an entire chapter to this topic; see Chapter 20 when you are at that stage.

CHAPTER SUMMARY

1. A caregiver is someone who takes care of another person who is sick or disabled, assuring a good quality of life for that person. The best caregivers offer and provide needed support while encouraging their patients to be as self-reliant as possible.

2. No one chooses to be a caregiver. Caregivers are responding to a situation that demands their attention and help.

3. Caregivers are a lifeline to patients with Alzheimer's and other dementias.

4. Caregivers are vital decision-makers regarding treatment, and are the doctor's partners in implementing a treatment program.

5. If caregivers don't take time to care for themselves, they may be at risk of becoming patients themselves.

6. There are distinct stages of caregiving, each with its own challenges.

Chapter 2

Different Kinds of Caregivers: Spouses, Other Family, Friends

CAREGIVING can be a very demanding and stressful activity, and because it can last for extended periods of time, you wouldn't want to take it on except for someone you love or to whom you are deeply committed. So for the most part caregivers will provide care only to someone really close to them: a spouse or partner, a sibling, a parent or parent-in-law. Occasionally someone will become a caregiver to a really good friend. In any case, a strong commitment to the person for whom you are going to provide care is absolutely necessary.

I have said that no two Alzheimer's patients are alike and by the same token no two caregivers are alike. For certain purposes, however, it may still be useful to draw some distinctions between different types of caregivers, based on the caregiver's relationship to the person for whom care is provided. Becoming a caregiver to someone changes your relationship to your loved one, depending on what your relationship was before the illness. Thus becoming a caregiver to your spouse differs from becoming a caregiver to your mother or your father.

Spouses as Caregivers

It can be assumed that spouses are very committed caregivers. They may have been together for forty to sixty years and thus have a huge number of experiences in common. At some level they have been caring for each other all along but both spouses have been contributing to this task. Now, however, a major shift in responsibilities is happening, with the patient passing on more and more of his or her household and personal tasks to the other person. While the caregiver for the most part is willing to take on these new responsibilities, there will be times when either the patient or the caregiver will experience anger or guilt over this life change. Caregivers, despite their best efforts, may get angry over the amount of responsibility that has been shifted to them. Or they may experience guilt from time to time, thinking that perhaps they are not doing enough, or that they lost their cool the day before. Patients too may get angry at the caregiver because they are losing prerogatives that they have long enjoyed, or they may feel guilty for burdening the caregiver excessively.

Adult Children as Caregivers

When an adult child takes on the caregiver role, the practical, emotional, and financial aspects of caregiving should be discussed among any siblings, particularly if only one of them is doing the bulk of caregiving. For instance, more than one of the children may contribute financially to the task. Another aspect to be considered in deciding which role each of the adult children will assume is whether any are in a "sandwich generation" situation, in which he or she is still very actively involved in child-rearing activities.

Role reversal is probably the most common change experienced by adult caregiving children as they take on a parenting role vis-à-vis their father or mother. This too can give rise to anger and guilt on both sides. Note too that because children have no "natural" authority over a parent, legal documents (like the power of attorney and related documents discussed earlier) will need to be executed early on in the disease in order to transfer this responsibility and authority to the caregiver.

Friends, Neighbors, or Distant Relatives as Caregivers

People who take on the caregiver role for persons with whom they have been less intimately connected prior to the caregiving experience seem to have a somewhat easier time, perhaps because they approach their task more clinically and objectively. They seem to experience extreme feelings of guilt and anger much less frequently than those with a long history with the patient, and they seem to come to the task more open-mindedly than caregivers who are closely related through blood or marriage. Perhaps for the same reasons, they also seem to find it easier to leave the caregiver relationship, which when it happens is clearly not to the patient's advantage.

Long-Distance Caregiving and Care Managers

Most caregivers of Alzheimer's and other dementia patients live either in the same household or in the same community. But sometimes there is no one nearby to provide care, and caregiving has to be done long-distance. It should be obvious that this kind of situation involves entirely different challenges and requires entirely different strategies. In particular, distance will almost always involve a *care manager*. Care managers are paid professionals who usually do not provide direct care to patients but instead coordinate the care of other personnel, usually the staff of an assisted living facility or another form of residential care. They work primarily on behalf of long-distance caregivers. Perhaps a brief case history will illustrate some of the elements of long-distance caregiving.

George and Emily Anderson lived in Philadel-phia, where he was employed by a prominent pharmaceutical firm. When he retired they decided that they would move to the west coast of Florida. Almost as if anticipating future developments, they were hesitant to leave the Philadelphia area, because two of their adult children lived and worked in nearby New Jersey, and they enjoyed visiting with their adult children and their grandchildren. But they moved anyway, looking forward to warmer weather and life in a coastal community.

Some three years later George died suddenly of a heart attack combined with a fatal cardiac arrhythmia. Their daughter Anne came down to Florida to help her mother deal with the funeral arrangements and help her get settled into a life of widowhood. She was assured that her mother could continue living independently, because her health appeared to be good. Anne returned to New Jersey, but maintained frequent telephone contact with her mother.

About two years later, however, Anne became concerned when her mother could not recall a previous conversation they had had. She asked her mother if she was all right, and her mother assured her she was "just fine." But there continued to be gaps in her mother's memory, and Anne finally flew down to Florida to see her mother and assess the situation firsthand.

What she found astonished her. Her mother appeared somewhat disheveled whereas she had previously always been immaculately groomed and dressed. When Anne opened the refrigerator in her mother's kitchen she found it stuffed with leftovers and smelling of spoiled food. On the table in her mother's breakfast nook she found an accumulation of newspapers that were weeks old. The garbage, too, apparently had not been taken out for weeks. Anne called her husband and her employer to tell them that she would be staying in Florida for a few days "to sort things out." Of course her first thought about a cause was Alzheimer's disease.

Anne quickly arranged for her mother to visit a local memory disorder clinic. She learned there that her mother was indeed suffering from the early stages of Alzheimer's disease, and could no longer live alone safely. A social worker in the clinic put Anne in touch with a senior care manager who helped her find a suitable assisted living facility and agreed to take on the supervision of the mother's care, with Anne being available by telephone as needed. For the most part this plan worked relatively smoothly.

Anne returned to Florida several more times over the next few months to see her mother, to consult with the care manager, and to arrange for an elder care lawyer to draft a durable family power of attorney and healthcare surrogate documents for her signature. Over the next several years this long-distance caregiving continued until Emily's disease became more advanced and she was admitted to a special memory care unit in a local nursing home. The same care manager continued to monitor the mother's progress "on the ground," with occasional return visits to Florida by Anne. Emily died peacefully about two years later.

CHAPTER SUMMARY

1. Caregivers vary in their approaches and feelings about their new role based in part on their relationship to their patients. Spouses and adult children, for example, each have unique needs and capabilities as caregivers. And unrelated or distantly related caregivers tend to have more objective, less conflicted relationships with their patients, though they may also be less likely to stay in the caregiving role.

2. In long-distance caregiving, care managers generally arrange and supervise care but do not personally provide hands-on care for patients; instead these tasks are often handled by care facilities or home health professionals.

Chapter 3

Why Alzheimer's Disease Demands Caregiving

W HY WOULD someone you love and feel so committed to need a caregiver? How did this someone lose the ability to care for him- or herself? No, this loved one didn't suddenly become lazy, or take on airs and demand to be treated like a prince or a princess. He or she was just living life in all innocence, and then something happened: Alzheimer's disease or another form of dementia. And these debilitating illnesses *demand* caregiving more than many other medical conditions do, for several important reasons.

Alzheimer's Is Relentlessly Progressive

Because Alzheimer's is a progressive disease, the affected person cannot simply make a one-time adjustment to his or her condition, but must make continual adjustments as abilities such as memory, decision-making, and self-care slip away one by one. A caregiver has to deal with the same changes, but the caregiver's capacities, if anything, grow rather than diminish over the course of the disease.

Alzheimer's Can Require Decades of Care

Although neither the caregiver nor the patient can predict exactly how long this disease will last, it is generally known to endure for two to twenty-five years. Caregivers can ask the patient's doctor about the expected rate of progression and duration of the disease. For more on how the rate of progression can be estimated by an experienced memory specialist, see Chapter 8.

Alzheimer's Affects the Brain

Since Alzheimer's disease attacks the patient's most vital organ, the brain, the disease will affect widespread areas of functioning, including memory, general intellectual abilities and decision-making, self-care, and the capability to manage one's emotions and behavior. Only a consistent, devoted caregiver will be able to deal with all these changes over the extended time during which they occur. Furthermore the caregiver will have to respond to increasingly complex and difficult demands by the patient as the disease changes the affected individual from a fully capable person to someone with a number of growing deficits, finally to the point where the patient is a mere shell of his or her former self.

CHAPTER SUMMARY

1. Alzheimer's is a relentlessly progressive disease that can last anywhere from two to twenty-five years.

2. Alzheimer's affects the person's most vital organ, the brain, and therefore has widespread effects on many functions.

3. The job of caregiving becomes increasingly more complex as the disease advances.

Chapter 4

Preparing for the "Job" of Caregiving

I T HAS BEEN found useful to think of caregiving as a "job." When caregiving is understood in this way, it becomes clearer to others and yourself just how much of your time will need to be devoted to this activity, and how adding it will limit other activities you are or have been carrying out, including paid employment or dealing with your household, your spouse, or growing children. Caring for someone with Alzheimer's disease may require that you renegotiate your responsibilities in these other areas with a boss, members of your own immediate family, or others.

In truth, caregiving has many but by no means all of the characteristics of traditional jobs. For instance, it is certainly hard work. It requires a set of skills for which some training is necessary. It has its own rewards. Yet what it does not have is regular hours nor does it produce any income—though it can preserve income since by doing the work of a caregiver you are avoiding the expense of hiring professionals.

What Kind of Training Is Needed?

While child rearing resembles caregiving for a disabled adult in some ways, the differences between them are enormous. For this reason caregivers need to learn the specifics of how Alzheimer's disease affects individuals and to acquire the training and preparation required for the specific responsibilities they will take on, responsibilities that will change as the patient's disease progresses. And while it is certainly true that no two Alzheimer's patients are alike, there are certain commonalities that, if understood, can help prepare caregivers for what they may need to deal with next.

Join a Caregiver Support Group

One of the strongest recommendations that I have for you is to join a caregiver support group as early as possible in the course of caregiving. To start your search for such a group, ask the doctor caring for your loved one where such a group exists and where it meets. Or better yet, if you are attending a memory disorder clinic, the clinic itself may conduct such a group. Failing that, inquire about a support group at your local chapter of the Alzheimer's Association or your local Area Agency on Aging, or look for an Alzheimer's caregiver support group in your community by conducting an internet search on your preferred browser. See the Appendix for more resource ideas.

Read All You Can about Alzheimer's Disease

One of the first caregivers I met taught me an important lesson. Harry had brought his wife, Eleanor, for an evaluation of her memory problems. He came into my office carrying a heavy briefcase that virtually bulged at the seams. After the formality of introductions I could hardly wait to ask what was in his briefcase. He told me and showed me: inside was a collection of articles, reprints, and photocopies filled with information on Alzheimer's disease. I was very impressed and since then I have recommended that caregivers familiarize themselves with available information about the disease, its treatment options, outcomes, and so on. You would do well to follow Harry's example. Fortunately today there is even more such information available than there was twenty years ago.

Find and Attend Caregiver Classes

Next, I would recommend that you locate a caregiver class. At the Suncoast Gerontology Center at the University of South Florida we teach such classes on a quarterly basis, covering all major aspects of Alzheimer's disease and caregiving. These classes are provided at no cost, and allow individuals caring for dementia patients to come repeatedly and ask questions. Those who attend more than one class often comment how much more they learned the second or the third time around.

Where can you find such a class? Many memory disorder clinics now conduct such classes. They may also be offered by the local chapter of the Alzheimer's Association or by long-term care facilities specializing in memory disorders.

On-the-Job Training, with Buddy Backup

As with most jobs, the most significant skills acquisition will come from on-the-job training. This will go on throughout your caregiver career. As new situations emerge you will need to refine both your knowledge base and your skills, based on what works and doesn't work for you with your particular patient. And while you can continue to learn from published reports and from the internet, your most valuable information will probably come from meetings with your caregiver group and with your doctor. I have one other recommendation to make: recruit a caregiver buddy, that is, someone whom you can call on day or night to ask for advice and to openly express your feelings. You will in turn make yourself available to your buddy in the same way. How do you find such a buddy? It may be someone you will meet in a caregiver group, or it may be your closest friend or one of your adult children, but it will definitely be someone who is familiar with your caregiving situation. Having such a confidante is enormously supportive and, in my view, a virtual necessity.

Other Tools of the Trade

There are a few other tools of the trade that you will want to develop. And if you are not naturally gifted with these tools, you and your patient will be well served if you can develop them to the level of a fine art:

1. **Patience, patience, patience.** Time and again you will find that nothing works as well as patience with your loved one who has been humbled and traumatized by Alzheimer's.
2. **A sense of humor.** If you can laugh it off, it will be so much easier to bear, for you and for your patient. I want to make sure you understand that I am talking about laughing *with* your patient, not *at* him or her. I will try to illustrate this approach with examples throughout the book.
3. **Cheerfulness.** A cheerful approach will smooth out many of the rough spots you will encounter in your caregiving. You may well ask how you can possibly manage to be cheerful in such a drastic situation. Part of the answer is to continue to nourish yourself by maintaining friendships and pleasurable activities that refresh and restore you.

Taking "Vacations"

Just as paid employment usually has benefits such as taking a vacation, you may also need to schedule breaks from caregiving to attend other vital functions in your life such as a family wedding, a graduation, or other such events. Or you may just need to schedule time away so that you can return to the caregiving task with renewed vigor and enthusiasm. You will learn that it is possible to do this by arranging for another family member to assume care for a week or two, or by arranging respite care with a special memory care facility that can look after your loved one for a week or up to a month while you attend to your own priorities and well-being. And there is no need to feel guilty for taking time out for this vital self-care; in fact, many patients truly enjoy being cared for by someone else, and are then especially delighted to be reunited with their regular caregiver.

CHAPTER SUMMARY

1. Although there are ways in which caregiving is and is not like a job, understanding it in this way can help

make clear to others and yourself the effects of this decision on other aspects of your life.

2. To prepare for the challenges of caregiving, be sure to join a caregiver support group, read all you can about Alzheimer's disease, and seek out and attend caregiver classes.

3. You will also learn a great deal from "on-the-job" training.

4. It can be very helpful to partner with a caregiver buddy.

5. Don't forget to use other valuable "tools of the trade," including patience, humor, and cheerfulness.

6. Plan to take "vacations" from your caregiver job, for your benefit and that of your patient.

Chapter 5

The Rewards of Caregiving

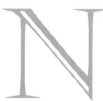EARLY everyone has some idea of how challenging and stressful it can be to provide care for an Alzheimer's patient. Having observed caregivers at close range over the last thirty years, however, I have also learned that caregiving comes with many rewards.

Caregiving Is Lifesaving

Individuals with more than mild Alzheimer's disease literally could not survive without a reliable and dedicated caregiver. As their self-care capacity diminishes and their capacity to judge declines, there are simply all too many ways that they would not be able to manage on their own. They could not take their medications by themselves, or safely drive a car or use other means of transportation. They could not handle their financial resources on their own. People with this disease absolutely require the affection and emotional support that only a devoted caregiver can provide. As the caregiver, you can feel happy knowing that you are not only doing a good deed, but are also a lifesaver for the affected person.

Alzheimer's has been described as a "monster" disease, and rightly so. It inflicts many cruelties and humiliations on affected individuals, and it does so over a long period. But having a reliable and attentive caregiver can ameliorate many of the worst effects and thereby make the Alzheimer's experience if not comfortable, at least tolerable. Knowing this should fill you, the caregiver, with enormous pride. You are truly making a huge difference.

Caregiving Is an Act of Unconditional Love

Your loved one may or may not be able to appreciate what you are doing for him or her. But providing care and love with or without reciprocation is the very essence of unconditional love, and being able to give such unconditional love is one of the most elevating of human feelings. It truly is better to give than to receive. Understanding this will help you get through those times when your acts of providing care are not valued but are met with anger and resentment. You must then remember that it is the disease that is speaking and not your loved one. One illustration of this is the experience of a caregiver I came to know through my practice:

> Jonathan is an eighty-year-old caregiver whose wife, Phyllis, has been in a nursing home for the past two years. Every morning he visits the nursing home to have breakfast with her. He continues to do so even though he realizes she no longer knows who he is. One day a friend asked Jonathan why he kept visiting Phyllis even though she no longer recognized him. Smiling, Jonathan patted his friend on the shoulder and said: "She doesn't know me, *but I still know her.*"

Jonathan's reward was in giving love, not in receiving it. Here is another illustration of how unconditional love works:

> Henry and Jane were divorced after some twenty years of marriage when Henry took up

with a younger woman. Jane watched from afar and saw Henry's new relationship fall apart. When Henry developed Alzheimer's disease on top of the diabetic condition that he had had for some years, the younger woman was nowhere to be found. As Jane saw Henry's disease progress to the point where he could no longer care for himself and would need to go to a nursing home, Jane moved back in with Henry and cared for him, saving him from an early admission to a nursing home, or from coming to harm from inadequate care. When asked why she was doing this, she just shrugged her shoulders and smiled. Maybe it was her way of rising above her husband's unfaithfulness, or maybe it was in honor of the love they had shared for a long time.

Caregiving Can Connect You to Others Who Understand

As I mentioned earlier, you should make every effort to join a caregiver support group early in the course of your caregiving career. There you will learn that you are not alone in your situation, and you will be welcomed into a new friendly and supportive community.

From the more experienced members of the group you will learn many techniques for dealing with various behaviors and situations. As you become more experienced, too, you can pass on to others techniques you have learned in your caregiving. As this next example shows, you may even form new friendships that will last you the rest of your life.

Helen, Marion, Martha, and Edith all belonged to the same caregiver support group. Each had a husband who was experiencing a different stage of Alzheimer's disease. Each of the four women came from very different backgrounds and would likely never have met each other in the ordinary course of social interactions. But somehow they developed a common bond, called themselves "the gang of four," met outside of the support group, and long after their caregiving days were over, kept up their friendship as each of them went on to experience differing illnesses and other life challenges. Whereas before they were there to support their husbands and each other, now they were there to support each other, finding an unexpected reward in their earlier shared tragic experience.

As a Caregiver You Will Discover New Strengths

As you rise to the challenge of helping someone with Alzheimer's disease time and time again, you will see yourself grow by leaps and bounds. You will grow in self-confidence. You will grow in creativity and innovation, gradually and perhaps imperceptibly. You will acquire a far higher level of patience, and you will be called on to use your sense of humor more often than you ever would have imagined.

Caregivers Are Helping to Defeat Alzheimer's Disease

Many of you will have the opportunity to contribute to our understanding of Alzheimer's disease, an understanding that eventually will lead researchers and doctors to solve the problem altogether. You can contribute to "a world without Alzheimer's disease" in a variety of ways. You can advocate with your political leaders for more research funding for Alzheimer's. One woman I know organized a new caregiver group in her church. Another woman did volunteer work for the Alzheimer's Association. One gentleman organized a brain donation network to foster research on the disease. Several men and women banded together in a retirement community to raise funds for providing up to three hundred hours of respite care at no cost to those in need. Many of you will share what you have learned about caregiving to teach "newbie" caregivers how to deal with various situations as they arise. Here is yet another illustration of how one woman made her contribution:

Anita's mother suffered from Alzheimer's disease. She sought out the best available treatment for her mother, moving her clear across the country so that she could participate in an experimental study with a new medication for the treatment of Alzheimer's. While her mother benefited from the new drug, she nevertheless went on to eventually die from the disease. Grateful for the care provided to her mother, Anita donated a large amount of money to the research center with which she had worked, establishing one of the first endowed research chairs on Alzheimer's disease. Not only did she make a major financial contribution herself; through "the power of the example" she inspired several other families to join her in funding the endowed chair. The several scientists who occupied the endowed chair went on to discover additional medications and treatment approaches that eased the burden of the disease for thousands of other patients in the center's service area as well as throughout the country. Anita had made a real difference in the battle against Alzheimer's disease.

Each of you will have differing opportunities to contribute, according to where and how you are situated. But you all are already contributing to our society by taking on the caregiver role for your loved one.

To be sure, caregiving for someone with Alzheimer's disease is one of the hardest jobs anyone will ever face. Yet caregiving has to be done—by someone. And if you have chosen to take on this challenge, however much you give to this job, you will also be amply rewarded.

CHAPTER SUMMARY

1. Caregiving is literally lifesaving for the patient, and it can "tame" or ease the most difficult symptoms of Alzheimer's disease and other dementias.

2. Caregiving is an act of unconditional love.

3. As a caregiver you will meet other caregivers who will enrich your life as you will enrich theirs.

4. As a caregiver you will be challenged like you have never been before, and as you rise to the challenge you will develop skills and discover inner strengths.

5. Caregivers everywhere are contributing toward the creation of a world without Alzheimer's disease.

PART II

Learning about Your Loved One's Condition

Chapter 6

Milder Forms of Memory Impairment

BEFORE discussing in detail the most serious types of memory impairment, such as Alzheimer's disease and other types of dementia, I would like to spend a little time explaining milder forms of memory impairment and how they differ from these more severe forms. There are two types of relatively mild memory problems that can happen to people in their sixties, seventies, and eighties: benign forgetfulness and mild cognitive impairment.

Benign Forgetfulness

Benign forgetfulness happens now and again to most people over age sixty-five. It is annoying but not serious.

Benign forgetfulness is characterized by a minor slowing of your memory capacity and manifests itself in a number of little ways such as forgetting where you parked your car or recognizing someone at a social gathering but being unable to recall his or her name right then and there. (A little while later the name may come back to you, making you feel somewhat foolish.) Or it may be a matter of having more difficulty in learning new information: learning how to operate new gadgets or remembering new phone numbers may not be as easy as it was years ago.

With a little extra concentration, these problems can usually be overcome. You may need to write down new information; you may need to make associations between familiar names or words and an unfamiliar word or name you are trying to learn in order to better remember it. You may have to have someone show you more than once how your new iPhone or DVD player works. But you can still learn, and you can still remember; you may just have to work at it a little harder. You may need to write yourself more notes, jot down the aisle number where you parked your car, or always place your house keys, your purse, or your wallet in exactly the same spot every time you come into the house.

The good news about benign forgetfulness is that it doesn't get any worse, and it does not lead to Alzheimer's disease. The disappointing news is that it doesn't get any better, either. You need to understand it, accept it, and adjust to it.

Mild Cognitive Impairment

Mild memory impairment, or more formally, *mild cognitive impairment,* or *MCI,* is a serious but not fatal disorder. It is characterized by completely forgetting whole sequences of events in which you have actively participated. Actually, "forgetting" is not an accurate description of what takes place. It happens because the event is never recorded in one's memory. This can be embarrassing, or worse. For instance:

> John, age seventy, lived in Florida and regularly went to an annual family reunion in Tennessee. Last year, when he came back, his son-in-law asked him about the reunion. John said he had not attended at all. But his daughter, who also attended, had recorded a videotape of the reunion. When John saw the video, clearly showing him participating and interacting at

the event, he broke into tears. He realized fully for the first time that he had no memory about the event. He also realized the implications of the occurrence: his memory problems were far greater than mere absentmindedness.

What happens in minor cognitive impairment is that the brain participates in the actual experience but no memory trace is laid down. It is somewhat like not pressing the "enter" or the "save" button on your computer. If such a situation occurs more than once or twice, the person should undergo a thorough memory evaluation by a specialist in memory disorders, that is, someone beyond your primary care doctor. This could be a psychiatrist, a neurologist, or an internist, but in any case, it should be a doctor who has a strong interest and extensive experience in memory evaluations. Standard memory tests may need to be performed. In addition, the person's ability for *delayed recall* of information may need to be tested. Problems with delayed recall—that is, recall of information that has just recently been presented—is one of the earliest signs of mild cognitive impairment. Further evaluation may require a session with a trained neuropsychologist, an MRI (magnetic resonance imaging) scan, or a PET (positron emission tomography) scan. An MRI is a test that produces an actual image of the brain, and it can pick up early indications of brain cell loss. A PET scan is similar but even more specialized and expensive, and it can detect changes in brain cell activity or metabolism before there is any loss of brain tissue.

If someone close to you is diagnosed with mild cognitive impairment, it can and should be treated by a memory specialist. Medications that have already been approved for the treatment of Alzheimer's disease, such as Aricept, Exelon, or Razadyne, have been shown in some cases to be of benefit to persons with minor cognitive impairment as well. Namenda has also been tried in mild cognitive impairment. While none of these medications have been approved for treatment of mild cognitive impairment, many treating physicians are using these medications in an attempt to keep the problem from progressing to full Alzheimer's disease or another form of dementia. This is still something of an act of faith, and the issue has not been fully resolved. In general, however, patients with mild cognitive impairment seem to not be harmed by treatment with one or another of these medications. With or without treatment, some one-half to two-thirds of patients with mild cognitive impairment progress to Alzheimer's disease.

CHAPTER SUMMARY

1. Benign forgetfulness is common in older persons and should not cause undue concern. New routines and strategies can be helpful in working around this problem.

2. Mild cognitive impairment is a more serious memory problem. If your loved one has more than one or two episodes of completely missing memories, a checkup by a memory specialist is recommended.

Chapter 7

Understanding
Alzheimer's Disease

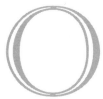NE OF the most frequently asked questions I receive from caregivers as well as from various healthcare professionals is: "What is the difference between Alzheimer's disease and dementia?" It is an important question. The short answer is that Alzheimer's is a specific type of dementia. Dementia, on the other hand, is any condition in which there is decreased memory, intellectual, and decision-making capacity due to the loss of brain cells in one or more regions of the brain. The loss of brain cells can be due to a number of specific diseases or conditions. These include specific diseases, such as Alzheimer's or Lewy body dementia; or it can be due to one or more strokes, single or multiple episodes of brain trauma; chronic alcoholism; toxins, such

as lead toxicity; or the result of a brain infection. Each of the dementias caused by different factors will produce a different pattern of diagnosis, progression, and treatment. The special characteristics of Alzheimer's disease will be discussed in the remainder of this chapter. The characteristics of the other forms of dementia, including vascular dementia, fronto-temporal dementia, Lewy body dementia, traumatic brain injury, and dementia associated with Parkinson's disease will be discussed in Chapter 10. In that same chapter I will also explain another type of memory problem called delirium. This is a *reversible* kind of memory problem associated with acute medical illnesses and sometimes side effects of medications, or with abuse or addiction to prescription medicines or so-called street drugs.

Characteristics of Alzheimer's Disease

So what is Alzheimer's disease? It is a disease of the brain whose cause is not yet fully understood. It typically affects people in their later years, through no fault of their own. It gradually takes over first a few areas of a person's life, then more and more areas. It is in fact a disease like no other. It affects about 5.2 million people in the United States at this time, and that number is going to double in the next twenty years. The reason for this is that more and more people live into their seventies, eighties, and nineties, and the prevalence of the disease increases drastically with each advancing decade. So although at age sixty-five only 1 percent of people have the disease, at age seventy-five 10 percent are affected, at age eighty-five some 35 percent are affected, and at age ninety this figure rises to 50 percent.

A Disease Like No Other

Some people have called Alzheimer's a monster disease, not only because it affects a huge number of people, but also because of what it does to those affected. It gradually eats away layer after layer of human functioning, starting with memory and decision-making capacity, and then into deeper and deeper layers of the personality. It attacks language, judgment, and the ability to communicate and care for oneself. Even more vexing than these losses is an accumulation of troublesome behaviors that increase gradually as the disease advances.

But patients with the disease are not the only ones affected. Caregivers of Alzheimer's patients also bear an enormous burden, especially as the disease progresses. And given the long duration of the disease, the total effect on the population is enormous—and growing. We have a veritable tidal wave of Alzheimer's coming our way, as a result of better medical care keeping people alive longer and into the age of greatest vulnerability. It would be difficult to overstate the magnitude of this disease.

Furthermore, beyond the suffering that the disease causes to affected patients and caregivers, it also places a monstrous financial burden on individuals, families, and state and federal governmental agencies. The current direct costs resulting from Alzheimer's disease are $214 billion, with a doubling of the cost expected over the next twenty years.

Effective caregiving is what humanizes this ordeal, both for the patient and the caregiver. Caregiving is what makes it possible to live with this disease rather than be overwhelmed by it. Family caregiving also vastly reduces the public or governmental cost of this disease.

Alzheimer's Disease Comes on Like Rain
in the Night

Alzheimer's disease comes on like rain in the night, imperceptibly at first, until it amounts to a flood that threatens to swallow both the patient and the caregiver. Let me give you a couple of illustrations of how this disease can sneak up on both patient and caregiver:

Pauline was a strong, independent woman who had been a bookkeeper and office manager all her working life, from her late teens. After her husband's death she had been a caregiver for her mother for many years. After her mother died, Pauline lived successfully on her own for a long time. Some health problems left her knowing she shouldn't live alone any longer and, with everyone's agreement, she had an apartment built onto the home of her younger daughter and son-in-law. With her own entrance, a mini-kitchen, space for card games with friends, and a dog and cat that visited any time, Pauline lived happily, actively, and comfortably for several years. A few minor memory hiccups occurred, but nothing that gave anyone a great deal of worry.

The daughter and her husband took an extended vacation and Pauline decided to spend that time at her older daughter's home. While there she mentioned she'd been having a little trouble balancing her checkbook. For her, this was really unusual—she prided herself on keeping her checkbook balanced to the penny. She didn't let her daughter look at the checkbook, however, saying she'd figure it out later. Then one day she asked her daughter to write a check for her (this daughter's name had been on the account as a secondary signatory for years) and the real problem was discovered. Pauline's checking account was in chaos—she'd been adding and subtracting the same entries multiple times and making mistakes with deposits and withdrawals, until her checking account was a complete mess and the funds were nearly gone.

The realization that their mother could no longer do math and could no longer keep her finances in order was a huge blow for her daughters. This was Pauline's field of expertise; this is what she had done well for nearly seventy years! This is when the family knew for sure that something more than "forgetting because you're getting old" was happening to their beloved mother.

Here is another illustration about the subtle onset of Alzheimer's disease.

Jim and Shirley were friends of ours, she an accomplished college professor, he a successful publisher. It was a second marriage for each of them. Perhaps this contributed to their both being slow to notice that something was wrong—each tended to pass off what was happening as just an adjustment to the new relationship. Jim began to forget conversations he had had with Shirley, which she wrote off as his simply being overly occupied with his work. Then Jim began to forget mutually agreed-on social appointments and became less attentive to his personal hygiene. Again, Shirley did not want to criticize Jim, because their relationship was still relatively new and she feared offending him.

It was finally his children who pulled Shirley aside and confronted her with the truth: Jim's forgetfulness and his need for reminders to take a bath or to change clothes represented a significant change in his behavior, and one that they felt needed medical attention. This was hard news for Shirley to accept, because Jim continued to be charming and socially competent, continued to use his erudite vocabulary, and continued to do the Sunday *New York Times* crossword puzzle without difficulty. But she heeded his children's concern and had Jim evaluated by a neurologist. The neurologist found problems with short-term memory and impairments with delayed recall of new information. He also ordered an MRI scan of the brain that showed atrophy in a small portion of the temporal lobe that serves memory. This news was shocking to both Jim and Shirley. They accepted the doctor's diagnosis of Alzheimer's disease, however, and followed his treatment recommendations. They continued to show their love for each other, and Shirley reluctantly came to realize that she would have to become the caregiver to Jim, brilliant though he was. Shirley consulted me both as a friend and as an expert on Alzheimer's disease, joined a caregiver support group, learned everything she could about the disease and about caregiving, and cared for Jim through all the stages of the disease, until he died some seven years later.

Alzheimer's Is a Brain Disease

It is important to realize that Alzheimer's is a disease, not simply a manifestation of old age. It is a disease in which brain cells die prematurely and progressively, leaving the individual with impaired memory function, impaired decision-making ability, and reduced reasoning and learning capacity. It is a very variable disease that can last anywhere from two to twenty-five years, eventually resulting in death, unless the person dies from another illness before then. President Ronald Reagan, for instance, lived with Alzheimer's disease for seventeen years.

In some individuals, Alzheimer's is primarily characterized by increasing degrees of memory and intellectual decline. Others with Alzheimer's may also exhibit behavioral problems, which can often be more vexing to the caregiver than memory problems. Behavioral problems can include depression, agitation, irritability, hostility, and even hallucinations and/or delusions. It is one thing to care for a nice little old lady who may be a bit forgetful but who is otherwise pleasant, and quite another to deal with a large, still-strong elderly person who is hostile, suspicious, aggressive, or fears that the caregiver is trying to poison him.

When Alzheimer's disease is suspected, the patient needs a prompt and definitive diagnosis, followed immediately by treatment in order to preserve as much memory and intellectual capacity as possible.

The Seven Warning Signs of Alzheimer's Disease

Now let me acquaint you with some of the hallmarks of Alzheimer's disease. I have called them the "Seven Warning Signs of Alzheimer's Disease," and they have been widely published by the Suncoast Alzheimer's and Gerontology Center at the University of South Florida and elsewhere. These signs have been helpful in alerting both lay persons and professionals to the possibility that Alzheimer's has taken hold. They are:

1. Asking the same question over and over again.
2. Repeating the same story, word for word, again and again.
3. Forgetting how to cook, or how to make repairs, or how to play cards—activities that were previously done with ease and regularity.
4. Losing one's ability to pay bills or balance one's checkbook.
5. Getting lost in familiar surroundings, or misplacing household objects.

6. Neglecting to bathe, or wearing the same clothes over and over again, while insisting that a bath was already taken or that the clothes are still clean.
7. Relying on someone else, such as a spouse, to make decisions or answer questions that one previously would have handled oneself.

The presence of two or three of these signs should alert you to the fact that a serious problem may exist. Four or five of these signs are definite signs of a major problem. And if all seven of these signs are observed, the person manifesting them almost definitely has Alzheimer's disease or another form of dementia.

Dementia is defined as any memory disorder due to the loss of brain cells. Alzheimer's disease is one of the causes of dementia. Other causes of dementia may include a major stroke or multiple smaller strokes, traumatic brain injuries, chronic alcoholism, or encephalitis. Dementia can also occur in the late stages of Parkinson's disease or as the result of Lewy body dementia, a variant of Alzheimer's disease (for more on dementias other than Alzheimer's disease, see Chapter 10).

If checking for the seven warning signs of Alzheimer's disease doesn't give you sufficient guidance, and you are still concerned about a family member or friend, there is another test available. At Duke University I developed the Short Portable Mental Status Questionnaire (SPMSQ; see Figure 1) to measure the presence and the degree of memory loss. The questionnaire is usually administered by a doctor, a nurse, or a social worker, but a layperson can do this as well. Accordingly, you could ask someone whom you are concerned about to answer these questions as a way of determining if he or she is experiencing significant memory loss. Please note that this is not a self-administered test. Further, although it allows the examining person to determine if the person's memory is normal, or whether he or she has mild, moderate, or severe memory loss, the test does not allow one to make a definitive diagnosis of Alzheimer's disease, or of any other memory-specific disorder. If there is evidence of significant memory loss, a full medical evaluation should be arranged as soon as possible.

Scoring of the SPMSQ

When evaluating the results of the Short Portable Mental Status Questionnaire, a score of none to two er-

SPMSQ

PFEIFFER
SHORT PORTABLE MENTAL STATUS QUESTIONNAIRE

INSTRUCTIONS: Ask the subject questions 1-10, record answer, and enter as "1" under appropriate column (correct/error). All responses, to be scored correct, must be given by subject without reference to calendar, newspaper, birth certificate or other memory aid.

Patient Name: _____

Date: _____

		CORRECT	ERROR
1.	WHAT IS THE DATE TODAY? Month_____ Day_____ Year_____ (Score correct only when the exact month, day and year are given correctly.)		
2.	WHAT DAY OF THE WEEK IS IT? Day_____		
3.	WHAT IS THE NAME OF THIS PLACE? (Score correct if any correct description of the location is given: "My home," accurate name of town, city or name of residence, hospital, or institution (if subject is institutionalized) are all acceptable.)		
4.	WHAT IS YOUR TELEPHONE NUMBER? (If none see 4A below) (Score correct when the correct number can be verified or when subject can repeat the same number at another point in question.) #_____ 4A. WHAT IS YOUR STREET ADDRESS? (Ask only if subject does not have a telephone.)		
5.	HOW OLD ARE YOU? AGE:_____ (Score correct when stated age corresponds to date of birth.)		
6.	WHEN WERE YOU BORN? Month_____ Day_____ Year_____ (Score correct only when exact month, date, and year are all given.)		
7.	WHO IS PRESIDENT OF THE UNITED STATES NOW?_____ (Only the last name of the President is required.)		
8.	WHO WAS THE PRESIDENT BEFORE HIM?_____ (Only the last name of the previous President is required.)		
9.	WHAT WAS YOUR MOTHER'S MAIDEN NAME?_____ (Does not need to be verified. Score correct if a female name plus last name other than subject's is given.)		
10.	SUBRACT 3 FROM 20 AND KEEP SUBTRACTING 3 FROM EACH NEW NUMBER ALL THE WAY DOWN. ___ ___ ___ ___ ___ ___ ___ (The entire series must be performed correctly in order to be scored correct. Any error in series or unwillingness to attempt series is scored as incorrect.)		

TOTAL NUMBER OF ERRORS [ ]

*ADJUSTMENT FACTOR

A) SUBTRACT 1 FROM ERROR SCORE IF SUBJECT HAS HAD ONLY A GRADE SCHOOL EDUCATION   [−]

B) ADD 1 TO ERROR SCORE IF SUBJECT HAS HAD EDUCATION BEYOND HIGH SCHOOL   [+]

TOTAL ADJUSTED ERRORS [ ]

SCORING KEY: 0-2 errors = intellectually intact; 3-4 errors = mildly impaired; 5-7 errors = moderately impaired; 8-10 errors = severely impaired.

INFORMATION OBTAINED BY:	DATE:

This form is also available online at www.DoctorEricKnows.com.

rors usually means normal memory function. A score of three to four errors suggests mild memory impairment. A score of five to seven errors indicates moderate impairment, and a score of eight to ten errors means severe memory impairment. The score only indicates the *severity* of the impairment, however. It does not indicate the specific cause of the memory impairment, and therefore cannot be used as a diagnostic tool. You will find a discussion of how Alzheimer's disease is diagnosed in Chapter 8.

When You Suspect Alzheimer's Disease

These days nearly everyone is at least somewhat aware of the possibility of Alzheimer's disease. We joke about it when we have forgotten a name or an event or where we parked our car, saying, "It must be my Alzheimer's kicking in." (By the way, Pfeiffer's law says that people only joke about those things that they are most serious about.) But Alzheimer's is no joking matter. If someone close to us used to remember things well, and now repeatedly fails to remember important information, we have every reason to worry that something serious is going on. If you observe one, two, or even three of the warning signs of Alzheimer's disease I have just discussed, your concerns should be heightened. What should you do next?

Continue your observations. Remain watchful for other signs of a faulty memory, of a lack of attention, or of an inability to complete a task your loved one has begun. If you see these signs, you will want to believe that they are not symptoms of Alzheimer's disease. But that would be denial. And although denial can protect us from pain or anxiety, it can lead us to ignore a problem that should not be ignored.

Denial can get in the way of your loved one's own perceptions about these changes, too. You might reasonably think that if you are beginning to see signs of memory loss, your loved one may also be aware of this change. But if denial is at work, or if the impairment is significant enough that your loved one doesn't remember having these glitches, he or she might not be ready to admit having a possible problem. Instead of being realistically concerned, the person may become irritable or depressed, or even become hypersensitive about being questioned in any way about whether and what he or she can remember.

This is the moment when you have to put into practice one of the cardinal lessons of caregiving: You have to be *so* gentle! Or to put it another way: Don't pounce!

Eventually, however, you may need to sit down with your loved one when both of you are relaxed and unhurried, and ask if he or she is aware of what you have noticed, and if it is causing any concern. If the answer is yes, you are well on your way to coming to grips with the problem, and the next step would be to schedule an initial medical evaluation with your loved one's primary care doctor.

If the answer is no, it will be more difficult for you to deal with this emerging problem. Your loved one may become quite defensive, irritated, or even accusatory, telling you that you are meddling in something that is none of your business. If this happens, it will be best to try to recruit allies, one or more other persons who have both you and your loved one's interests at heart, and to bring the matter up again a bit later, ever so gently. If none of this works you should discuss your concerns with your loved one's doctor at the next appointment. It can take weeks or even months, sometimes years, before the problem can be confronted by the patient and an evaluation can occur. Hopefully your persistent concern will be appreciated and acted on.

Preparing to Take on the Caregiver Role

Once you know that you are most likely dealing with Alzheimer's disease, it is time to get ready to take on the caregiver role. Keep in mind that when you become a caregiver it will be in addition to whatever else is going on in your life and whatever other obligations you already have. If this sounds heavy to you, it is. But doing anything new is difficult unless you learn all there is to know about the job. This includes two main goals: (1) Learning everything that you can about the disease you are dealing with in your loved one, and (2) Learning everything that you can about you, yourself, in the caregiver role. In the next several chapters, I will try to teach you everything you need to know so that you can fulfill both of these goals.

Patients with Alzheimer's Can Also Have Other Ailments

Just like others in the aging population, patients with Alzheimer's can have other diseases such as diabetes, hypertension, arthritis, congestive heart failure, and so on. This means that in addition to being an Alzheimer's caregiver you may also have to help your Alzheimer's patient manage his or her other ailments. I know you hadn't bargained for this. But unfortunately it, too, comes with the territory. This is particularly true as Alzheimer's disease progresses, as more and more of the tasks of managing the patient's other illnesses become yours to manage. Poorly controlled diabetes, hypertension, or heart disease—all will make the symptoms of Alzheimer's disease worse. In addition, Alzheimer's patients are more prone to have accidents leading to broken arms, a broken pelvis, or, even more seriously, a broken hip. These will not only add to your tasks in caregiving but may also worsen the patient's Alzheimer's symptoms, leading to, for example, greater confusion, anxiety, or depression. If you are going to provide care for your loved one's Alzheimer's disease, this means you will have to become the patient's general health care manager as well. As you read this, I can already hear you saying, "Thanks a bunch!"

Hospitalizations

Some patients with Alzheimer's disease find hospital visits very unsettling. Just being away from home, exposed to multiple strangers and strange procedures—not to mention the possible anesthesia or other medications added to or replacing the patient's usual medications—can throw them off. They are likely to become grossly disoriented, frightened, agitated, hostile, and delirious. Many such patients begin to hallucinate or to become delusional shortly after admission. The hospital staff may respond by placing such patients on powerful antipsychotic medications, but the side effects of these medications may make the situation even worse. Such complications can prolong the duration of the hospital stay, at considerable additional expense.

Accordingly care must be taken that patients with Alzheimer's disease be considered for hospital care only when it is absolutely necessary. An office visit or even a home visit by an accommodating doctor will be much less disruptive than hospitalization, and much less expensive.

We were really fortunate that Mama's Alzheimer's didn't create too many major behavioral problems in the first few years. She had been settled into her home with us for several years and felt comfortable and secure. That made my caregiving duties easier and also made it somehow a more loving experience for both of us. I had the caregiver job at home and my sister accompanied Mama to doctor's visits and handled her finances. We did end up bringing in people from an excellent home health care company for a few hours a day a couple of days a week. Unhappily, all that ended when a health issue cropped up and we and her doctor thought she needed to be hospitalized.

Mama understood the situation initially and was OK during the exam and check-in process. But in the hospital room she went into a panic, had to be restrained, and every attempt to calm her failed. Even the sedatives she was given reacted in the opposite way they should have; she slept very little and only when she was completely exhausted. Someone had to be with her the whole time; I only slept about 18 hours during the 60 hours she stayed in the hospital. It became painfully obvious that the Alzheimer's had accelerated and worsened while she was there and her doctor reluctantly told us it was very unlikely she'd be in a condition to return to our home and my care.

So we put her into a rehabilitation and nursing facility for a month in order to take the next step into an assisted living facility. The care was excellent but it was clear she was changed right from the first days there. From a woman who made sense in conversations, who laughed, who loved to do little puzzles and play her version of solitaire, who walked in the back-yard with our animals, she became vague, slow to speak, and uninterested in much of anything. The little puzzles she enjoyed only confused her and she'd just look up at me saying, "I don't know what that is."

Mama walked into the hospital holding my hand, smiling and chatting. She entered the assisted living facility in a wheelchair and without a word. The Alzheimer's had taken giant steps, carrying her farther and farther away from herself and from us.

This case history and others like it illustrate why hospitalization should be avoided, if at all possible, in favor of office or home care. But sometimes it can't be helped; when a hip fracture or other major medical incident occurs, a hospital is the necessary choice. If this happens, the patient's principal caregiver should accompany the patient to the hospital, and be there for as much of the stay as possible. The caregiver, as well as hospital staff, should continue to reorient the patient to the new setting, if need be, over and over again. Attempts at sedation often make the situation worse, and restraints applied to the patient can be perfectly disastrous. In addition, it is important for patients who have been on Alzheimer's medications that these medications either be continued in the hospital or be restarted as quickly as possible. (Alzheimer's medications are frequently discontinued when someone is admitted to a hospital.)

Some observers have noted that patients in the later stages of the disease, when they are much less cognizant of their environment, are less disturbed by being placed in a hospital. Nevertheless the need for hospital care for such patients should also be weighed very carefully.

Chapter Summary

1. It is essential to understand the difference between Alzheimer's disease and dementia.

2. Alzheimer's disease comes on almost imperceptibly, "like rain in the night."

3. Alzheimer's is a disease of the brain, not merely a manifestation of old age.

4. Know the "Seven Warning Signs of Alzheimer's Disease," and become familiar with the Short Portable Mental Status Questionnaire.

5. An Alzheimer's diagnosis should be made by a medical specialist, not a general practitioner.

6. There are steps you can take now to get ready to take on the caregiver role.

7. Patients with Alzheimer's can also have other diseases that will require their caregiver to become their general health care manager as well.

8. Patients with Alzheimer's disease or other dementias can find hospital stays upsetting.

Chapter 8

Advances in Diagnosing Alzheimer's Disease

I T USED to be said that the diagnosis of Alzheimer's disease could be made only by performing a brain autopsy. While this was a perfectly reliable way of making the diagnosis, doing so after the patient had already died did not benefit either the patient or the caregiver. Today, however, it is possible to make the diagnosis of Alzheimer's disease in the living patient with 90 to 95 percent accuracy. Moreover, the diagnosis can be made at every stage of the disease—mild, moderate, or severe. It can even be made when the patient has only mild cognitive impairment, which we now regard as either a forerunner of Alzheimer's disease or as its earliest stage.

The Importance of Obtaining a
Definite Diagnosis

Once you and your loved one have become aware that a memory problem has developed or is developing, it is very important that a definite diagnosis be established as soon as possible so that treatment can be initiated. Since becoming aware of a memory problem is certainly not welcome news to you or your loved one, it should not be surprising that both of you may wish to ward off acceptance of this fact by various forms of "explanations" and denial. You may say to yourself, "It is just old age" or "My husband (or wife) has just been working too hard." But if concerns continue, a full medical evaluation should be pursued.

While any number of specialists (such as a neurologist, geriatric psychiatrist, or internist) can make a valid diagnosis of memory problems, including of Alzheimer's disease, I recommend that you make an appointment at a full-fledged memory disorder clinic where a whole team of specialists is available to pursue whatever diagnostic procedures are needed. Too many individuals have simply gone to their family doctor, complained of memory problems, been asked to repeat three words after three minutes, and then been prescribed Aricept, being told that it is "just dementia." Don't go this route. Instead insist on a full evaluation and a prognosis, at a medical center that can offer the assurance that you and your loved one will be followed continuously for the entire duration of the illness.

Establishing a definite diagnosis of Alzheimer's disease is important for a variety of reasons. First, you as a caregiver need to know what you are dealing with. Second, a diagnosis is needed for patients to participate in any government-sponsored assistance programs for this particular disease, or to meet the requirements for certain facilities, or to participate in any clinical studies for Alzheimer's disease. Also, sometimes a doctor's written statement of the diagnosis can be a clarifying point for other family members not directly involved in the care of the patient. They can look at it and say, "Okay, now I know what is wrong." And in an odd way, having this clarification can be a great relief.

What Is Needed to Make a Diagnosis?

Only a doctor, preferably one who is a specialist in memory disorders, can make a definite diagnosis of Alzheimer's disease. In order to do so, the doctor will need all of the following items:

- A detailed history of how memory problems have developed, obtained from both the patient and the caregiver
- A thorough general medical history; a complete physical and neurological examination; and a battery of lab tests, including a complete blood count, tests of liver and kidney function and thyroid function, cholesterol and other lipid tests, a vitamin B12 level, and a fasting blood-sugar level
- A standard electrocardiogram (EKG)
- At least one imaging study of the brain, preferably an MRI scan, a computed tomography (CAT) scan, or even better, a PET scan of the brain
- An assessment of the degree of memory deficit, using one of the memory screening instruments such as the Folstein Mini-Mental Status Examination (MMSE) or the Pfeiffer Short Portable Mental Status Questionnaire (SPMSQ)

The doctor will also need, in some cases, a full-scale neuropsychological evaluation by a psychologist; and still more selectively, certain genetic tests and possibly measurements of amyloid beta 42 peptide and tau protein in the patient's cerebrospinal fluid, blood, or urine. Several of these tests require some additional explanation. For instance, when an MRI or CAT scan of the brain is performed, special care needs to be taken to investigate the appearance of the temporal lobe, particularly an area called the hippocampus and the amygdalar area. Atrophy, or shrinkage, in these areas is almost completely specific to Alzheimer's disease. In addition, when a PET scan of the brain is performed, additional information about the state of the brain will be obtained. A regular PET scan measures the amount of blood flow and glucose metabolism in the brain, especially in the temporal lobe where memory function occurs. Decreased blood flow and/or glucose metabolism is an early indicator of Alzheimer's disease.

A still newer, modified PET scan is now beginning to come into use: amyloid PET scanning. Amyloid plaques in the brain are the most reliable hallmarks of Alzheimer's disease. Amyloid PET scanning measures the amount of amyloid plaques in the brain; the number of amyloid plaques seen, especially in the temporal and the frontal lobes of the brain, is a measure of the likelihood and the severity of Alzheimer's disease. While this type of scan is currently used for research purposes, it is likely that in the near future it will become a more regular part of a diagnostic workup for Alzheimer's.

Note, too, that neuropsychological testing should be performed when the results of other tests are inconclusive, when the person is only very mildly impaired, or when he or she has a high level of education. Other, more specific lab tests are discussed next.

Laboratory Tests: Helpful, But Not Definitive (Yet)

There are several lab tests that can contribute valuable information to the diagnostic process, even though no definitive lab test yet exists for Alzheimer's disease. That is, these days the diagnosis of Alzheimer's disease is still a clinical process, even though in experienced hands it can be 90 to 95 percent accurate when compared with brain autopsy findings.

There are two major forms of Alzheimer's disease:

1. *Inherited Alzheimer's disease* accounts for less than 2 percent of all cases. This form of the disease generally starts in individuals in their forties, and patients with this form of the disease generally die in their fifties or early

sixties. The offspring of these individuals have a 50–50 chance of also developing the disease, and genetic DNA testing can reveal whether a child of such an individual has that gene.

2. *Spontaneous Alzheimer's disease* accounts for almost all other cases of Alzheimer's disease. This form of the disease begins only rarely when someone is in their sixties, and instead more commonly begins when the patient is in their seventies, eighties, and nineties. Age is the greatest risk factor for spontaneous Alzheimer's disease—that is, the risk increases with advancing age, and family history plays only a relatively minor role. But in these cases a genetic test, the ApoE test, may have a possible role to play.

You may not need to know all the details about the ApoE test, but if you or your doctor is considering using it as a diagnostic tool, it may be good to have this information (if the ApoE test is not at all being considered for your loved one, you may skip the rest of this paragraph). The ApoE test determines whether an individual has one or more of the genes that favor development of Alzheimer's disease. There are three variants of the ApoE gene: ApoE-2 is protective against Alzheimer's disease,

ApoE-3 is relatively neutral, and ApoE-4 favors the development of Alzheimer's. Each individual inherits one ApoE gene from his or her mother and one from the father. Carriers of one ApoE-4 gene have a slightly higher risk for developing the disease than do persons without any ApoE-4 gene. Carriers of two ApoE-4 genes have a significantly greater risk of developing the disease, estimated at almost 70 percent. Today the ApoE test is used primarily as a research tool, not as a clinically useful diagnostic tool. The reason for this is that people without any ApoE-4 gene can still develop Alzheimer's. More than half of those with two ApoE genes will develop the disease eventually. But the ApoE gene is only a *risk factor* for developing the disease and not a determining factor. Again the biggest risk factor for developing the spontaneous form of Alzheimer's disease is advancing age, not heredity.

Other types of lab tests exist that have some usefulness in the diagnostic process. These measure the levels of various chemical compounds relevant to Alzheimer's disease, either in the urine, the blood, or in cerebrospinal fluid. *Amyloid plaques,* made up of clumps of amyloid-beta 42 peptides, and *neurofibrillary tangles,* made up of tau proteins, are the most specific findings of Alzheimer's disease in the brain. Tests for levels of these compounds currently form the basis for the spinal fluid, blood, and urine tests for Alzheimer's disease. Currently the most sensitive test for Alzheimer's is a spinal fluid test for these chemicals: an elevated level of tau protein and a decreased level of amyloid-beta 42 peptides are found in patients with established Alzheimer's disease. Such a finding can support a clinical diagnosis of Alzheimer's disease, but by itself is not diagnostic. Tests that measure similar compounds in the blood and urine are also sometimes used to support a clinical diagnosis, but similarly are by themselves not definitive. In fact, most experts on Alzheimer's disease feel that such lab tests should at this point be used primarily as *research tools* and are not recommended for routine use in making a diagnosis of Alzheimer's disease.

What Caregivers Need to Know about the Diagnosis

Once your loved one has had a complete diagnostic evaluation, what parts of the diagnosis do you as a caregiver need to know? Here are the questions to which you should receive relatively clear answers:

1. Are you definitely dealing with Alzheimer's disease, or are you dealing with a different impairment, such as vascular dementia, or Lewy body dementia, or post-traumatic or post-encephalitic dementia?
2. Does your loved one have Alzheimer's disease as well as something else, such as vascular dementia?
3. If you are definitely dealing with Alzheimer's disease, what stage of the disease is your loved one experiencing now?
5. What will be the rate of progression: slow, intermediate, or rapid?
6. In addition to memory and intellectual impairment, are you also dealing with behavioral problems? These can be more troublesome than memory problems, and may require separate interventions.

You will need to know the answer to all of these questions so that you can make appropriate plans, both for your loved one and for yourself.

Chapter Summary

1. Only a doctor, preferably a specialist in memory disorders, can make a definite diagnosis of Alzheimer's disease.

2. As a caregiver, you'll want to know what is needed to make a definitive diagnosis of Alzheimer's disease, as well as the value and limitations of the various laboratory tests available for helping to diagnose it.

3. It is important to establish a definite diagnosis for your peace of mind, and to help you create a realistic and helpful care plan.

4. When a diagnosis is made, be sure to get all of your questions answered, for your sake and for the benefit of your loved one.

Chapter 9

Alzheimer's Disease Can Now Be Treated

A S RECENTLY as the 1990s there was no treatment for Alzheimer's disease. Real progress has been made in this area since then as a result of scientific research. Significantly, the treatments that have been developed should be started as soon as the diagnosis has been definitively established, since they basically help to ease symptoms and to slow the progression of the disease. Starting treatment as soon as possible, then, will give your loved one the best chance of preserving his or her highest possible level of function. Any delay in starting treatment will produce less favorable results, since the disease will have progressed further and the starting level of the patient's function will accordingly be much lower and the burdens on the caregiver that much greater.

The currently available treatments do not cure the disease, but like treatments for the vast majority of chronic diseases, they can help patients manage their symptoms. Just as a diabetes patient who undergoes successful treatment to control his diabetes still has diabetes, after effective treatment of Alzheimer's disease, the patient will still have Alzheimer's disease—but the symptoms will be less severe and the rate of progression will have slowed significantly.

Medications for Treating Alzheimer's Disease

There are now two classes of medication available for the treatment of Alzheimer's disease: cholinesterase inhibitors and NMDA inhibitors. Examples of cholinesterase inhibitor drugs are Aricept, Exelon, and Razadyne, whereas there is only one drug available, Namenda, that is an NMDA inhibitor. The two classes of drugs work by entirely different mechanisms, which means that when they are used together they can produce a greater benefit than when either category of drug is given alone. For example, the combination of Aricept and Namenda was shown in one study to produce greater benefit in terms of memory function, self-care capacity, and disruptive behaviors than could be obtained with Aricept alone. The FDA has approved the use of Aricept, Exelon, and Razadyne for mild and moderate Alzheimer's disease, while Namenda has been approved for moderate and severe Alzheimer's disease. Aricept has also been approved for continued use into severe stages of Alzheimer's disease.

Treatment should be begun as soon as the diagnosis has been made. Your doctor will probably recommend starting with one of the cholinesterase inhibitors in the mild stages, and adding Namenda in the middle (moderate) and late (severe) stages. Treatment with these medications should probably continue until late into the disease.

These medications are not a cure, but they can at first improve and later on slow the progression of memory problems, of self-care capacity, and of disruptive behaviors. Combination therapy with these medications can also help the patient to maintain his or her communication skills.

In addition to medications for treating the symptoms of Alzheimer's disease, work is also going forward on seeing whether nutritional products such as Axona or palm oil can improve symptoms. The idea is that ketones may be used by brain cells as an alternative fuel to glucose when glucose utilization has become impaired. Vitamin supplements, including folic acid, vitamin B12, vitamin B6, and vitamin E, have also been found useful in some studies, although not everyone agrees about the findings and what they mean.

Intense research efforts are currently under way to test several new medications that work in novel ways and offer new approaches to combating Alzheimer's disease. These newer medications may be able to bring about additional benefits and further slow the progression of the disease, so it will be important for you to watch for announcements of such additional breakthroughs. You may also wish to enroll your loved one in a clinical study of experimental medications. The value of participating in clinical studies is discussed in greater detail in Chapter 11.

The medications mentioned in this section may also be of value in treating the symptoms of other forms of dementia, even though none have been specifically approved for this purpose by the FDA. If you are caring for someone struggling with another form of dementia, be sure to explore the best available medications with your loved one's memory doctor.

"Smart Pills"

Any discussion of treating the symptoms of Alzheimer's disease quite naturally evokes curiosity about whether the medications used to treat it could also be used to prevent Alzheimer's disease, or whether they can be used by healthy individuals as "smart pills" to improve their intellectual abilities. At this time there are no solid data to support the use of these drugs for either of these "off-label" purposes. A few studies have shown some benefits to college students of using these drugs to prepare for exams or to test pilots who use flight simulator machines. I recommend waiting for further clarification of these issues, and for further safety testing in normal, healthy individuals, before trying any of these medications on your own.

Managing Behavioral Symptoms

Many Alzheimer's patients do not show any significant behavioral disturbances, especially in the early stages of the disease. As the disease progresses, however, a variety of troublesome behavioral symptoms will make their appearance. These may include mood disturbances like sadness, depression, apathy, and negativism or refusal to eat; disruptive behaviors such as agitation, verbal and/ or physical aggression; wandering; sleep disturbances, including day-night reversals; hallucinations and delusions; and more. In later chapters I will discuss the more phase-specific behavioral problems and outline management approaches to them. For now I just wanted to make you aware of them as possibilities as well as to let you know that this book, your loved one's memory doctor, and members of your caregiver support group will all help you to deal with them. In addition, you'll want to know that there are medications available that your doctor can prescribe for severe and or specific behaviors related to Alzheimer's disease. These include antidepressant medications for severe depression and major tranquilizers for severe agitation or for hallucinations and delusions.

Nonmedicinal Approaches

There are also a number of nonmedicinal treatments available for Alzheimer's disease. These can include memory-training classes, especially in the early stages of the disease. Vigorous physical exercise has also been proven to be remarkably beneficial in improving memory as well as behavioral problems.

The Most Critical Part of Any Treatment Program: You

By far the most critical component of any treatment program for someone with Alzheimer's disease or any of the other dementias is you, the caregiver. An informed, trained, and committed caregiver is what is needed most. The remainder of this book is devoted to helping you become that caregiver. And to the extent that I do not cover everything that you will need to know or do, I will refer you to additional resource persons or organizations.

How Long Will You Need to Provide Care?

Alzheimer's disease is an extremely variable disease. It can last anywhere from two to twenty-five years. So how long will you have to provide caregiving support to your loved one? While no one can give you a precise answer to that question, it is possible to come up with a good estimate based on careful observation of your loved one by you and the medical care team. For instance, if your loved one has reached only the mild or early stages of the disease after a few years, then one can judge that he or she is pursuing a slow course, and that the entire illness may last anywhere from fifteen to twenty-five years. If your patient has already reached the severe stages in two to three years from start of the first symptoms, however, then he or she may be expected to run the entire course of the illness in as little as four to five years. Most commonly, however, the entire course of the disease can take from seven to ten years, from first symptoms to final outcome. Hopefully this knowledge will help you prepare yourself mentally and practically for what lies ahead.

CHAPTER SUMMARY

1. Alzheimer's is now a treatable disease, though there is still no cure.

2. There are medications available for easing the symptoms of Alzheimer's disease, including behavioral symptoms, and it is important to keep paying attention to developments in how medicines are being used,

alone and in combination, to help Alzheimer's patients. Nonmedicinal treatments are also available.

3. You might consider participating in clinical studies in Alzheimer's disease, to help researchers achieve a cure faster, and to give your loved one the opportunity to try new treatments earlier.

4. The most important element in any treatment plan for Alzheimer's is you, the caregiver. Given the progression of your loved one's symptoms, it should be possible for a memory specialist to predict how long you may need to be a caregiver.

Chapter 10

Other Forms of Dementia, and Delirium

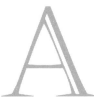 LZHEIMER'S disease is by far the most common cause of dementia, accounting for approximately 65 percent of all cases. But a number of other conditions can also cause dementia. Each of these tends to produce somewhat different patterns of memory loss and disordered behaviors, although from a caregiver's point of view tending to the needs of these patients is in many ways like caring for someone with Alzheimer's disease. Here I will discuss only the most common other forms and causes of dementia—that is, vascular dementia, mixed vascular and Alzheimer's dementia, Lewy body dementia, fronto-temporal dementia, and post-traumatic, post-encephalitic, and post-alcoholic dementia. In general these are distinguished from Alzheimer's disease

by both their effects on memory and their behavioral manifestations. To determine which kind of disorder is at work, brain images using MRI or PET scans are almost always needed. These scans then require careful interpretations by radiologists thoroughly familiar with these disorders.

Vascular Dementia or Post-Stroke Dementia

Vascular dementia is the second most common form of dementia, after Alzheimer's disease, and accounts for approximately 15 percent of dementias in the older population. It is the result of one or more cerebrovascular accidents, either one or more strokes or multiple mini-strokes. Contrary to Alzheimer's disease, its onset is sudden and/or stepwise, with some recovery occurring after each such episode. The end result after multiple small or larger strokes may be very similar to what is seen in Alzheimer's disease, however: severe memory loss, loss of self-care capacity, as well as speech impairment, loss of sensation, or muscle weakness, depending on where the cerebrovascular damage occurred in the brain. MRI scans are particularly useful in establishing the diagnosis of vascular dementia, because MRIs are

good for showing where in the brain a stroke has occurred as well as the size of the affected area.

From a treatment perspective the most important
aspect of caring for such patients is attention to cardiovascular and cerebrovascular risk factors. Accordingly
such patients need to be under the care of an experienced internist or cardiologist, as well as a memory specialist. The goal is systematically to reduce the risk of
additional strokes by lowering high blood pressure, con-
trolling diabetes, and treating irregular heart rhythms.
Lifestyle changes may also be indicated. In particular,
weight loss needs to be achieved in those who are significantly overweight, a regular exercise program needs
to replace a sedentary lifestyle, and reliable measures
for reducing stress need to be taught and practiced. If
additional cerebrovascular events (strokes) can be prevented, the course of dementia in such patients need
not be progressive. In fact, if your loved one works dili-
gently on his or her post-stroke rehabilitation, in some
cases memory function, speech, and muscular function
can actually improve.

Although no medications have been specifically approved by the FDA for memory problems due to vascular dementia, the medications currently available for

the treatment of memory problems in Alzheimer's disease can sometimes be helpful; ask your patient's doctor for details.

Mixed Vascular and Alzheimer's Dementia

Since both Alzheimer's dementia and vascular dementia are relatively common in an elderly population, both types of dementia can coexist, resulting in a different set of symptoms and progression of each disease. If your loved one has both conditions, it will be essential to try to reduce his or her cardiovascular risk factors with the same vigor as is necessary for the treatment of vascular dementia. This mixed form of dementia may account for some 5 to 10 percent of dementia cases.

Lewy Body Dementia

Lewy body dementia differs from Alzheimer's dementia in a number of ways. In terms of brain pathology, it is characterized by the presence of dense inclusion bodies, so-called Lewy bodies, located in the cortex of the brain and in certain areas of the brainstem that control locomotion.

I should let you know up front that Lewy body dementia is a far more difficult disease to manage than Alzheimer's disease, from both a caregiver's as well as a physician's point of view. Like Alzheimer's disease, Lewy body dementia is a progressive disease, with symptoms worsening over a matter of years. As in all dementias, there are progressive memory and intellectual deficits. In addition, persons with this disease typically experience fluctuating levels of consciousness and awareness coupled with hallucinations, primarily visual hallucinations, and Parkinson's-like muscular stiffness and tremors. As a result of the stiffness and tremors these patients may experience multiple falls, transient episodes of unconsciousness, and disturbed moods, especially depression. Hence my earlier warning that caregivers will need to deal with a striking multitude of altered states and behaviors, and must seek treatment from the patient's physician for whichever symptoms are most prominent. This will include medications used in Alzheimer's disease for memory problems, major tranquilizers for the treatment of hallucinations and delusions, and medications typically used in Parkinson's disease for the treatment of muscular stiffness and tremors. In most cases the course of Lewy body dementia is more rapid than in Alzheimer's disease, and may require residential or nursing treatment earlier than in other forms of dementia.

Dementia Associated with Parkinson's Disease

Parkinson's disease is a kind of neurodegenerative disease characterized by changes in muscle control. Its symptoms include tremors, unsteady gait, slow muscle movements, and stiffness of the facial muscles, which causes a lack of facial expression and a low voice volume. In the middle and later stages of Parkinson's disease most patients experience some degree of memory deficit or dementia. Usual treatment of Parkinson's disease includes medications such as L-dopa, with or without carbidopa. Parkinson's disease patients are generally treated by neurologists. When dementia is also present, the memory-enhancing drugs used in Alzheimer's disease, such as Aricept and Exelon, can sometimes improve memory function.

There is an interesting reciprocal relationship between Parkinson's and Alzheimer's disease: late in Parkinson's disease, symptoms of dementia develop in perhaps 15 percent of such patients, and late in Alzheimer's disease, Parkinson symptoms develop, again in perhaps 15 percent of such patients. In addition, in a small number of individuals both diseases may occur simultaneously, which then worsen the overall disability experienced by the patient, and may cause a somewhat more rapid progression of all related symptoms.

Fronto-Temporal Dementia

Fronto-temporal dementia is yet another variant of dementia. It is characterized by a loss of brain cells in the frontal and temporal lobes. Any particular patient's symptoms are determined by where exactly the brain cell loss occurs. As with all dementias, there is progressive memory loss, though sometimes not as severe as in Alzheimer's disease. Patients also usually experience an impairment of social inhibitions and decorum, impulsivity, as well as a decline in "executive function" (the ability to carry out complex actions that require discipline and planning). The disease may be more prominent on either the right side of the brain or the left side. People with left-sided forms tend to show more social disinhibition and impulsive behavior, whereas those with right-sided versions of this disease seem to struggle more with language and word formation.

Highly successful treatments have not yet been established for this type of dementia. The typical memory-enhancing medications used in Alzheimer's disease have not been much help. Other so-called psychotropic medications (anti-anxiety, anti-depressive, or anti-psychotic medicines) also have few positive effects in these patients. This means that a lot of the burden of managing these patients' behavior falls to the creative ingenuity of their caregivers. Special caregiver support groups for caregivers of patients with fronto-temporal dementia can therefore be especially valuable, because caregivers can learn successful behavioral interventions from more experienced caregivers. Distracting the patient with a new focus of attention, praising or complimenting the patient for his or her appearance or for more appropriate or helpful behavior, and involving the patient in a new or established pleasurable activity—all have proven to be successful strategies with these patients.

The onset of fronto-temporal dementia is usually somewhat earlier than that of Alzheimer's disease, that is, between fifty-five and seventy years of age, and it lasts generally ten years or less.

Post-Traumatic, Post-Encephalitic, and Post-Alcoholic Dementias

Sometimes single or multiple episodes of trauma to or toxic exposure of the brain leave behind permanent damage. In general, the disorders that result—post-traumatic, post-encephalitic, and post-alcoholic dementias—are not progressive but vary based on the severity and frequency of the trauma, or the nature of the toxin. (Exceptions would be chronic alcoholism or work-based exposure to toxins, which would progress if the exposure to alcohol or another toxin continued.) Typical causes of post-traumatic dementia are exposure to explosions on the battlefield, or having had multiple head traumas and concussions when playing sports such as football, hockey, and boxing. Given these causes, patients with post-traumatic dementia tend to be younger than those suffering from other forms of dementia.

Early-Onset (Hereditary) Alzheimer's Disease and Genetic Risk

Sometimes caregivers become concerned about the possibility that because someone else in their family has experienced Alzheimer's disease, they themselves are at greater risk for developing it. This concern is for the most part unwarranted. Advancing age is the greatest risk factor for developing Alzheimer's disease. For example, at age sixty-five only 1 percent of individuals have Alzheimer's. At age seventy-five this has risen to 10 percent. At age eighty-five some 35 percent of such individuals have the disease, and at age ninety, nearly 50 percent are affected by the disease. Having a single blood relative with Alzheimer's disease increases the risk for developing the disease only slightly.

Some 2 percent of patients with Alzheimer's disease, however, have a strictly hereditary form. In these cases the onset of symptoms occurs in people's forties and fifties, and generally runs a more rapid course, often causing death within seven to ten years. Generally there is a history of at least one parent who had Alzheimer's disease, since the children of these individuals have a 50 percent chance of also getting the disease.

The takeaway message here is that hereditary factors do not play a major role in determining whether someone may be at risk for developing Alzheimer's disease unless two or more blood relatives have had the disease or that person is related to the rare 0.5 percent of Alzheimer's patients who suffer from a clearly inherited form of the disease. Genetic testing is available to determine which child or children have the genes causing Alzheimer's disease. This leads to the difficult ethical as well as practical questions of whether and when such children ought to be tested. Given the importance of the answers to such tests, I would advise that such families receive genetic counseling before proceeding with testing for hereditary Alzheimer's disease.

Prevention and Treatments for Non-Alzheimer's Dementia

To the extent that the devastating condition of dementia can be avoided, we all need to take care that we, and our loved ones, are doing our best to avoid injuries and exposures to environmental toxins. The U.S. military as well as professional sports associations have recently become increasingly aware of the potential brain-damaging effects of explosions and repeated concussions, among other injuries. With political and social pressure, we can hope that industrial awareness of toxins and adequate mental health treatments for addictive disorders such as alcoholism will also follow.

In terms of treatments, the memory-enhancing drugs approved for Alzheimer's disease are generally effective in easing the symptoms of these other forms of dementia. Anti-depressant and anti-anxiety agents may also be useful when your loved one is suffering from depression or anxiety.

If your loved one is experiencing one of these other forms of dementia discussed in this chapter, you will want to familiarize yourself with as much information about that particular form of dementia by asking your doctor for available literature on that topic, or undertake your own search for information by going to www .WebMD.com or www.Google.com. In addition, please be aware that despite the differences in caregiving pointed out in this chapter, many of the challenges of caring for any dementia patient are still very similar to those experienced by someone caring for a loved one with dementia due to Alzheimer's disease.

What Is Delirium?

One other type of memory disorder, delirium, is quite different from both Alzheimer's disease and other forms of dementia. Delirium is a condition of the brain in which brain cells are temporarily impaired due to metabolic or toxic conditions, or in the course of an infectious illness. Symptoms of delirium include impaired memory, confusion, changing levels of consciousness, and sometimes vivid hallucinations and/or delusions. A number of metabolic diseases can cause delirium, such as poorly controlled diabetes or a failure of the heart, kidney, or liver. Most infectious diseases accompanied by high fever, such as pneumonia, can also cause delirium. Finally, delirium can also be caused by the overuse or dangerous mixing of medications, alcohol abuse, or the use of illegal and so-called recreational drugs such as Ecstasy, alone or in combination

In order to identify the cause of delirium, the patient needs a complete medical evaluation that includes documenting any history of associated symptoms such as pain, cough, or exposure to known infectious agents. The doctor must also obtain a meticulous history of any recent change in prescription and over-the-counter medications, as well as complete information on any drug addiction or abuse.

Delirium caused by a medical illness will generally resolve once the underlying illness is treated successfully. In case of multiple medications or overmedication, a change in drug regimen is in order. In case of drug abuse or addiction, not only is abstention from further immediate use required but rehabilitative treatment also needs to be begun as soon as possible. Almost by definition, delirium is always potentially reversible unless the patient succumbs to his illness or dies of an overdose. In fact, because delirium can also occur in patients who are already suffering from a degree of dementia, occasionally an underlying dementia condition will first be recognized when the patient's mental state doesn't return to normal after being treated for delirium.

CHAPTER SUMMARY

1. A number of forms of dementia other than Alzheimer's dementia exist, and of these, vascular dementia is the most common and Lewy body dementia is the most complex.

2. Post-traumatic forms of dementia affect mostly younger people, especially men.

3. Early-onset (hereditary) Alzheimer's disease makes up only a small portion of patients with dementia.

4. Dementia can also be associated with the later stages of Parkinson's disease.

5. Taking care to avoid injury and environmental exposures

can help prevent the occurrence of other types of dementia.

6. Even though there are significant differences among other types of dementia and between these other types and Alzheimer's disease, caring for such individuals can be in many ways like caring for Alzheimer's patients.

7. Delirium is quite different than dementia: it is a reversible kind of mental impairment often caused by medical illnesses or medications.

Chapter 11

The Value of Participating in Clinical Studies

LINICAL studies, also called clinical trials, are the way that new medications are tested for effectiveness. These studies are an essential part of the process of determining which drugs should be approved by the Food and Drug Administration (FDA) for general use. For this reason they are important to pharmaceutical companies, the FDA, and the general public. But did you know that they can also be of great value to caregivers and their patients? Clinical trials allow patients to experience the benefits of potential new medications long before they become generally available. Furthermore, if you can enroll your loved one in a clinical study, both of you will experience a multitude of positive results:

- You both will become part of a caring family, the clinical research team.
- Your patient's memory problems and overall medical care will be followed far more closely than if only an individual physician were in charge.
- You will have access to clinical study personnel to answer questions, and you will receive suggestions as well as emotional support throughout your participation in the study.
- The new medication may indeed provide greater benefits than the currently available medications alone. In addition, you and your loved one will be considered pioneers in the battle against Alzheimer's disease.

Clinical studies are being conducted in multiple research centers across the United States, perhaps near to or in your community. You can locate such studies by searching on the internet and entering the phrase "Alzheimer's disease, clinical studies." Your doctor may also be aware of where these studies are being conducted, or you can contact your local chapter of the Alzheimer's Association for this information. Participation in most clinical studies is at no cost to the patient or caregiver. Some studies even provide reimbursement for the cost of travel to the site. But not everyone can participate—your loved one may not be eligible depending on the stage of the disease, other illnesses, or other medications he or she is taking.

Possible Drawbacks

There are also some potential disadvantages to participation in clinical studies. First, clinical studies are generally "randomized, double-blind, and placebo controlled." This means that your loved one may be on a placebo (inactive) medication for a portion of the time he or she is participating in the study. Neither you nor your loved one, not even members of the research team, will know during the study whether or not the active medication was given. In addition, since medications in these studies have not yet been approved for this use, there is the possibility of adverse side effects. Be assured, however, that patients in such studies are very closely monitored for the occurrence of any side effects.

On the whole, the advantages of participating in clinical studies far outweigh any of the disadvantages, for the two of you, and for the community at large. If you complete a clinical trial, you and your loved one may have the distinction of making a real contribution to discovering a new treatment for Alzheimer's disease.

CHAPTER SUMMARY

1. There are many benefits to participating in clinical studies, for both you and your loved one. There are also some potential drawbacks.

2. On the whole, the advantages of participating in clinical studies far outweigh any disadvantages.

Chapter 12

The Future of Research and Treatments

T HE MEDICATIONS we currently use to help patients with Alzheimer's disease only modify the *symptoms;* they do not cure or modify the course of the disease. What these drugs do is to correct some of the neurotransmitter abnormalities seen in Alzheimer's disease. Specifically, drugs like Aricept, Exelon, and Razadyne raise the level of the neurotransmitter acetyl choline, which is low in Alzheimer's disease. The drug Namenda decreases the level of glutamine in the brain to correct the excess of glutamine seen in Alzheimer's patients. Neither of these categories of medications can stop brain cells from dying. Therein lies the challenge for researchers from here on in: to discover or synthesize medications that actually attack the underlying causes of Alzheimer's disease and other forms of dementia, thereby leading to, if not reversal of the disease, at least a halt to its progression.

To understand the difference between symptom treatment and curative or disease-modifying treatments, let us look at a more easily understood example: infectious disease. Medications like aspirin, Tylenol, or Aleve can treat the *symptoms* of a bacterial infection, such as pain and fever. Only an antibiotic, however, such as penicillin or a tricyclic antibiotic, can eradicate the bacteria causing the infection. In a sense, then, researchers are looking for the "penicillin" to cure Alzheimer's disease, not simply another "aspirin" or "Tylenol" to improve the symptoms of the disease.

The Search Continues

For the past ten years researchers have been testing what is called the "amyloid theory" of Alzheimer's disease, which assumes that excess beta amyloid in the brain causes brain cells to die. Double-blind studies of medications that reduce amyloid in the brain, however, have not resulted in either memory improvements or a slowing of the disease process, so researchers are now close to abandoning this theory. Instead the search is now on for other factors that actually cause brain cells to die. One of the new theories driving this search implies that inflammation in the brain causes brain cell death. This means that agents that prevent or reduce abnormal inflammation in the brain are considered possible prospects for medications to help people with Alzheimer's disease.

We now know as well that the disease starts perhaps fifteen to twenty years before clinical symptoms become apparent. Diagnostic tests available today, specifically amyloid PET scans, will allow people at risk for the disease to be identified earlier and earlier, before irreversible loss of brain cells has occurred. Individuals with parents who have or had Alzheimer's disease, or persons who have more than one close blood relative with the disease, would be selected for such testing, as well as individuals who have a known genetic predisposition for developing Alzheimer's disease. This would include persons with two copies of the ApoE-4 gene or of other genetic markers still to be identified. Those individuals with amyloid deposits on PET brain imaging could then begin to receive the disease-modifying treatments well before clinical symptoms of memory loss occur, thereby preventing the disease from ever becoming a clinical problem.

Cooperation Is Now Driving Research

I am pleased to report that the search for disease-modifying treatments for Alzheimer's is now intensifying, as evidenced by several new developments at the highest level of decision-making. In 2013 President Obama allocated an additional 100 million dollars to the U.S. National Institutes of Health for research on the disease. At the international level, Prime Minister David Cameron of Great Britain chaired a G-8 meeting to discuss international cooperation on Alzheimer's research. And perhaps most amazingly, most of the major (usually very competitive) pharmaceutical companies have signed agreements for joint funding and sharing of research findings among themselves and with the U.S. National Institutes of Health. Together they have announced two very ambitious goals: achieving the ability to *prevent* the disease by the year 2020, and gaining the ability to *stop* the disease by the year 2025. All of us can now hope that these goals will be accomplished.

The Promise of Disease-Modifying Treatments

Once disease-modifying treatments for Alzheimer's disease become available, the entire landscape of care and treatment for those affected by the disease will change dramatically. The role and responsibilities of family caregivers will be transformed—instead of handling day-to-day care and being their loved one's overall health care manager, they will be primarily concerned with identifying loved ones who might be at risk and assuring that they are tested and treated. In addition to reducing the enormous emotional cost on patients and caregivers, the huge medical costs and associated expenses incurred by individuals, families, and governments for treating and caring for Alzheimer's patients would also be greatly diminished. Truly it is in the interest of all concerned that we each do everything possible to foster and sponsor research that will lead to a "world without Alzheimer's disease."

CHAPTER SUMMARY

1. There is a major difference between treating the symptoms of Alzheimer's disease and treating its underlying cause or causes.

2. Disease-modifying treatments are not available yet, but the search is intensifying as research groups and pharmaceutical companies cooperate and share their findings.

3. Disease-modifying treatments for Alzheimer's disease hold enormous promise for reducing the physical, emotional, and financial costs for patients, caregivers, families, and the community at large.

PART III

PROVIDING CARE FOR YOUR LOVED ONE

Chapter 13

The Early Stages:
A Caregiver in Waiting

I N THE earliest stages of Alzheimer's, when both you and your loved one are still just trying to figure out what is happening, you cannot yet be called the "caregiver." Assuming the role of caregiver requires a delicate negotiation to establish that someone is in need of care, and that isn't at all clear early on. As I wrote earlier, "You have to be *so* gentle." Many an individual in the early stages of the disease has blurted out, sometimes with some degree of anger, "I don't need a caregiver." And for the most part they are right. At this stage the affected individual can still pretty much do everything he or she needs or wants to do: drive a car, make a telephone call, socialize, cook a meal, get dressed and ready in the morning. In fact, you are only a "caregiver in waiting," waiting to step in if you are needed, and not otherwise. You haven't been "commissioned" yet.

As it becomes clearer to both of you where help is needed, you can offer that help, and then again step back when nothing further is required. This kind of back and forth is likely to go on for weeks and months, as the diagnosis is pursued and established, and as the treatment is begun.

Working with an Elder-Law Attorney

Before getting into the specifics of working with an elder-law attorney, let us assume that your loved one has been evaluated by a memory specialist and that a diagnosis of Alzheimer's disease has been established. Let us further assume that this was done early enough and that the memory specialist has indicated that your loved one is only "in the early stage" of Alzheimer's and that a well-known test of memory function, the Mini-Mental Status Examination, or MMSE, yielded a score between twenty-one and twenty-eight. (If your loved one is already in the middle stage of the disease with an MMSE score between eleven and twenty, or in the late stage, with an MMSE score under ten, it may no longer be possible to draw up valid documents like the ones discussed in this section.)

This is now the time to consult with an elder-law attorney. Such an attorney can draft a number of critical documents that both you and your loved one will need in order to manage your financial and other affairs during the remainder of the illness. I specify the need for an elder-law attorney, because this is a very specialized field of law and many general, real-estate, or business and contract attorneys are not familiar with the complexities involved in dealing with progressive memory disorders. Working with an elder-law attorney early on in the course of the disease ensures (1) that the documents will hold up as legally valid, and (2) that the wishes of your loved one are adequately reflected in these documents. This may also be a time to add a second name to your or your loved one's checking account so that someone trusted is always available to authorize needed expenditures.

Durable Family Power of Attorney

Assuming now that it has been agreed that you are going to be the primary caregiver, one of the tasks to be accomplished is to have your loved one give you a power-of-attorney document. This document allows your loved one to make decisions for himself or herself for as long as he or she is able and then, when the affected person is no longer able to do so in the judgment of the treating physician, that authority will pass easily and automatically on to you. This seamless transfer allows you to make the household and financial decisions necessary to keep your loved one's care consistent and your own situation stable.

Healthcare Surrogates

You will also want to establish yourself and/or another trusted member of the family as a healthcare surrogate, that is, someone who can make medical-related decisions related to Alzheimer's or other illnesses throughout the remainder of your loved one's life. This may be the same person named in the power of attorney, or it could be someone else who has a more extensive understanding of the medical decisions that might have to be made.

A Last Will and Testament

This is also an excellent time to have your loved one review his or her will and to amend it, if necessary. If no will has been made, this is definitely the time to do so. You may well ask if someone with mild Alzheimer's disease can still make or amend a will. The answer is "yes," since in the early stages of this disease, someone with Alzheimer's is still capable of making a will or amending an existing will. This is so because the legal requirements for making a valid will are relatively simple. The person making a will must understand that he or she is making a will and that the making of a will generally relates to the distribution of the property and valuables after death; the person must also know and understand what is called in legal terms "the natural objects of their bounty"—in other words, who his or her family members and close friends are, and whether those persons are whom the person wishes to bequeath part or all of his or her possessions. The third requirement is that the person understands the nature and location of the properties, valuables, and other belongings.

Because wills of persons with Alzheimer's disease are often contested on the basis that the person no longer understood what he or she was doing or that undue influence was used to obtain a specific will provision, the fact and circumstances of a will being drafted or amended by a person in the early stages of the disease should specify how and where the will was made, who was in attendance, and that there was medical certification that the person was still capable of making a such a will or amendment to the will. "Undue influence" is said to have occurred when a patient is "persuaded" to make a change in his or her will or to make other concessions to benefit the caregiver under some sort of threat—perhaps that the patient will be placed in a nursing home or otherwise will no longer be cared for by that caregiver. Of course such threats are terribly unethical and immoral, and proof of such undue influences will invalidate any such change or provision in a will. It is generally viewed as a situation in which a weakened mind is influenced under duress to make a decision favorable to the caregiver.

After the early stages of Alzheimer's diseases, it is advisable that no new wills be created and that no significant amendments to an existing will be made. This advice is in keeping with the general recommendation that wills be made and amended in a timely fashion, when all physical and mental capabilities are still intact.

It should not be too surprising that bringing up these subjects may stir up some initial resistance or anxiety, not only in your loved one, but in you, the caregiver, as well. But these are absolutely vital steps you will need to take together with your loved one. If you take these steps gently and patiently, waiting for some acceptance and understanding before proceeding, you will have the best chance for making this an emotionally comfortable process for both of you.

Anticipating Together the Changes to Come

During the early stages of this disease it should be your goal to keep life flowing in as normal a way as possible, although both you and your loved one know that change has come and that more change is coming. Exactly what that means will, of course, depend on how you have been living your lives together up to this time. It may evoke in you or your loved one a desire to take an inventory of all that you want to do while it is still possible: take a cruise, see Europe, spend time with the grandchildren. This could be the time to fulfill a dream or create your own "bucket list." (If you are not familiar with this term, it means deciding what you still want to do, separately or together, before either one of you "kicks the bucket.") In the case of Alzheimer's disease it is not so much a matter of before either one of you dies, but before one of you becomes so disabled that certain activities might no longer be possible. Again, this is a very delicate exploration. The mutual love and trust that has been built between you and your loved one will make this as easy as possible under the circumstances.

An Alzheimer's Diagnosis: Should Your Loved One Be Told?

Should your loved one be told that he or she has a diagnosis of Alzheimer's disease? This is indeed a very important question, but one for which there is no easy answer. You as the caregiver should certainly know that you are dealing with Alzheimer's. But for the affected individual, the answer is not so clear. In my medical practice, I did not have a hard and fast rule about it, but rather was guided by the circumstances of each particular case. If patients asked me whether they had Alzheimer's disease, I generally asked what they knew about the disease and whether they thought they had it. Some individuals would be extremely threatened by hearing this diagnosis applied to them, and in those cases I usually told them that they had "a memory problem," that I was very interested in helping them with their problem, and that we have medication to treat memory problems. I would also tell them that they may have to rely on other people, their spouse, their children, and so on, to help them with certain decisions and activities. If the patients appeared to be capable of accepting the Alzheimer's disease diagnosis, I would tell them that they "probably" have Alzheimer's disease, leaving a ray of hope that it just might be something else. The reason for handling this issue with a certain degree of discretion is that some individuals have a really negative, scary view of what Alzheimer's disease is. Occasionally someone has even attempted suicide after being told of the diagnosis, without having been given the information about treatments available and how to live with Alzheimer's. But one way or another, the affected person must be told that he or she has a serious memory problem, and what the implications of that might be, including the availability of treatment and support.

If Your Loved One Is in Complete Denial

If your loved one is unwilling or unable to admit that any change is coming, that is, if he or she is in complete denial, the job of working together to take the next best steps becomes a lot harder. I have seen quite a few people, particularly people who are or have been powerful and prominent in their communities, reject any admission that something is wrong. If this happens, both the patient and the caregiver are in real trouble. In this scenario, your loved one won't avail himself or herself of the treatment that is needed, and preparation for the future will not take place. I myself have been involved in a number of cases where total denial that anything was wrong made it impossible for a powerful person to ever be evaluated, much less treated, for Alzheimer's disease. In my experience this level of denial is more common among men than among women, and among individuals whose names are household words for the contributions they have made to their communities. Their previous accomplishments, however, only make the results of their denial all the more tragic. Let me illustrate with a few examples:

Harmon was a very successful developer of sub-divisions and other major real estate projects. He attracted ample funding for his projects and drew similarly accomplished partners to work with him. His successes allowed him to fund numerous initiatives that helped his community: a swimming pool in a low-income neighborhood, a facility for victims of domestic violence, and a major beach restoration project. His wife was the first to notice serious and worsening memory lapses, which he completely denied. His partners then began to notice that he missed appointments and miscalculated the funding for new projects. Their pleas for him to seek help were met with hostility, and eventually this led to the departure of several of his partners. His entire enterprise reached the point of near collapse. His wife had come to the conclusion that he suffered from Alzheimer's disease. She was aware that some treatments were now available, but she could do nothing to persuade him to seek help. She was unwilling to have him declared incompetent in a court of law, given his prominence in the community and the negative publicity that this would involve. She came to see me on a number of occasions to discuss her plight. I offered her some advice on coping techniques for some of his behaviors. His illness continued to progress until he could no longer care for himself and he was admitted to a nursing home in the advanced stages of his disease. It was very painful for me to see the damage done to one of the most brilliant minds in the community, and the pain this caused his loving wife. Harmon died about a year after being admitted to the nursing home.

Unfortunately this was not the only case in which I was unable to be of any help to a patient prominent in the community, and only of limited service to his wife, who was never officially "allowed" to be a caregiver:

Jeremy was a brilliant attorney in one of the most powerful law firms in his community. He had political ambitions as well as skills, and was elected to the Congress of the United States. He served for five full terms, or ten years, before his memory problems became apparent to his family and to his staff. He denied that there was any problem with his memory and refused all efforts of help. He retired from Congress during his sixth term, citing his wish to be with his family more of the time as the reason for his decision. His wife was utterly frustrated. I saw her on several occasions. Apart from offering her sympathy and understanding, there was again little that I could do. The stigma of admitting to Alzheimer's disease was still too great, even after President Ronald Reagan had acknowledged his disease publicly.

I cite these examples in the hope that a greater awareness of the damaging effects of a patient's denial will keep this tragic scenario from playing out in other families.

Becoming an Official Caregiver

Now that you have been told that your loved one has Alzheimer's disease, and your loved one has more or less accepted that he or she either has a serious "memory problem" or "probably" has Alzheimer's disease, you are ready to step into the caregiver role officially. During these early stages of the disease, the demands made on the caregiver are relatively modest. Patients are still able to communicate effectively with their caregivers, and they are able to perform all the basic as well as the more complex activities of daily living (eating, dressing, grooming, making purchases, using public transportation, driving an automobile, using the telephone, and so on). When it comes to short-term memory, however, their performance falls short. They may forget appointments, they may not be able to deliver a message they took over the phone, they can no longer manage their money, and they may forget to take their prescribed medication. So what is needed is a kind of a hovering caregiver who allows the patient to do what he or she still can do, but is also ready to step in and provide assistance when it is needed. In other words, the number of hours you will actually be doing specific things for your loved one will be relatively few, but your role as a watchful "guardian angel" will be in operation 24/7. Yes, caregiving really is the quintessential 24/7, or 24/7/365, job. This is the time to adopt the saying "accept what you cannot change" as your personal mantra. It will help you to maintain your balance, and you will be using it a great deal for quite a while.

Now take a deep breath! We have a lot more to cover.

Caregiving Is a Job: It Requires a Plan and a Schedule

It may be useful to think of caregiving as a kind of job. You have to take it seriously, you have to plan, and you have to have a schedule. It is not like any other job; remember 24/7/365? So what do you do first, and what do you do next, and what do you do after that? Good questions, though they're not so easy to answer.

To start with, you need to be a keen observer. Look for what has been changing or is changing, and then decide if there is something you need to do about it. Not all changes you may see will require a specific response. To help organize your observations, you might want to look for likely changes in five areas: (1) memory, (2) communications, (3) routine everyday activities, (4) mood, and (5) behavior.

Caregiving Requires a New Point of View

Before discussing how to deal with the changes I just mentioned, I need to let you know that two changes in attitude and point of view at this point can make a huge difference in how things go between you and your loved one. The first is to try to assume a clinical attitude toward whatever happens between you and your patient. Strange as it may seem, I am recommending that you try not to deal with your loved as a spouse or a parent or sibling and instead respond as if you were an unrelated health professional dealing with an illness. This way it will not feel so much like your mother or your husband or your wife is refusing to do something or yelling at you, but rather a patient for whom you have assumed responsibility.

Another needed change is to respond to behaviors not from your own point of view, but from the patient's point of view. For instance, if your loved one asks the same question over and over again, it will help immensely if you understand that from the point of view of the patient he or she is asking a new question every time. If your loved one does not remember your neighbor's name, or that he or she had breakfast a scant two hours ago, understand that from the patient's point of view the familiar neighbor is a total stranger, and he or she has absolutely no recollection at all of having had breakfast just a few hours ago. Remember: you have to be *so* patient!

Dealing with Changes in Memory

During this phase of the disease you are likely to discover that memories of recent events or recent conversations, and updating of events or times, will start to deteriorate noticeably. You may find yourself having to repeat conversations you have had, or you may need to answer the same question more than once. And your loved one may not be able to keep track of the day of the week and the date, since these require constant updating.

You may want to keep the day of the week and the date displayed somewhere prominently in your home to help with orientation. If your loved one does make mistakes, it is important that you respond *calmly* rather than with annoyance.

Dealing with Changes in Communication

You may notice that your loved one is unable to finish a sentence, or may get stuck on trying to find a word that simply won't come out. If you understand enough of the sentence, you don't need to do anything. If you can guess what word your loved one is trying to say, go ahead and supply the word, so that the conversation can continue. For example: if your loved one says "We have to go to the . . . (can't come up with the name)," go ahead and say "Williams's house" so that your loved one can complete the sentence. This will be less frustrating for both of you than if you wait for the right name to emerge.

Changes in Everyday and Self-Care Activities

Let us say your spouse starts to mow the lawn or to wash the dishes, but doesn't finish the job. There is no need to make a big deal out of it. Ask your spouse to please start again on the same task (remember: you have to be *so* gentle!) or finish the job yourself.

You will also notice a tendency on the part of your patient to be less attentive to grooming and changes of clothing. Men may go without shaving for several days. The best way to respond to that is to ask the man to shave for special occasions, such as going out to dinner or visitors coming to the house. Both men and women tend to change clothes less regularly. These changes are best responded to by gentle reminders and increased tolerance for such behavior.

At this stage of the disease, problems with regard to toileting tend to be relatively mild also. Here the word "prompting" will become very important to you. The person generally still has full control of bodily functions such as getting to the bathroom on time. If there is an occasional accident, a regular regimen of reminders or of taking the patient to the bathroom every two to three hours can minimize the problem. But this will become an area of much greater concern in the middle and late stages of the disease. One thing you might do at this stage is to move your loved one's bed closer to the bathroom, and orient it so he or she can see the bathroom when getting up.

Changes in Mood or Behavior

Behavioral problems are generally quite mild at this stage of the disease. They tend to stem from the fact that your loved one is quite aware that he or she is not functioning as well as earlier. There may be some mild depression or irritability, or a lack of interest in initiating or completing activities. A generally loving and supportive attitude toward the patient will alleviate many of these relatively minor problems. If you notice your loved one becoming blue or irritable, try to initiate a new shared activity. Suggest something that you know he or she usually really likes to do, like "Let's go for a walk; it is such a beautiful day today," or "Let's have a picnic out in the back yard today." Or offer a compliment that you can sincerely make, such as "You're wearing such a nice outfit today," or "I sure appreciate your helping me put away the dishes." If more serious mood or behavior problems crop up, discuss them with the doctor or bring them up for discussion in your support group.

Making a Schedule for Each Day

You may wish to have a lot of variety in your life, but patients with Alzheimer's disease generally do not. It turns out that having a similar routine of activities each day works best for persons throughout the course of this disease. What that routine will consist of depends on what routines the person has followed before developing the disease. You might think that routines would become boring, but they can actually be quite comfortable. Routines around meal times are probably the simplest and most reliable to establish, so you might start there.

Plan Something Fun Every Day

Try to find an activity each day that both you and your loved one can enjoy. It could be a walk in the park, playing a game of cards, cooking a meal together, exercising together, playing with your dog or cat, going shopping for groceries, dancing, listening to music, watching a favorite video, or any number of other things. In our city, one of the theme parks allows people to purchase an admission ticket one time and to return as often as they wish throughout the year. Perhaps if a park or museum in your area offers a similar deal, you could visit repeatedly without spending a lot of money. Another activity that many patients with Alzheimer's disease enjoy is looking through photo albums of relatives and friends, or photos of an earlier period in your lives. If you yourself can't think of any such activities, talk to other caregivers about what is enjoyable for them and their loved ones. This brings me to one of the most important bits of advice that I can give you: if you haven't done so by this point, join a caregiver support group.

Join a Caregiver Support Group

As I mentioned earlier, joining an Alzheimer's caregiver support group will be a lifesaver for you. First of all, you will see that you are not alone in struggling with some of these problems. Second, you will have an opportunity to learn from other caregivers strategies that have worked with their loved ones. You will also enjoy the camaraderie of being with people who are in the same boat as you are. How do you find a caregiver group? The doctor or clinic to whom you are taking your loved one is likely to know of one. If not, you can call your local Area Agency on Aging, chapter of the Alzheimer's Association, or hospital to find out when and where such groups meet. You can even learn about caregiver groups by going on the internet, typing in "Alzheimer's support group" followed by the name of your community, and seeing if you find a listing there.

A caregiver group usually consists of a group facilitator who may be a memory specialist, a social worker, nurse, or doctor, or even a lay leader, as well as a dozen or more participants who are dealing with various stages of caregiving for their loved one. Generally there is no cost to attend. Sometimes a support group even has an activity program in which your loved one can participate while you attend the group session. Later on, when you yourself have become an experienced caregiver and have discovered some things that work really well with your patient, you will be able to pass on these "secrets" to other caregivers in the group. You will find that they will be very grateful to you for your advice.

Write about Caregiving

Many caregivers have learned that writing about their experiences and thoughts during caregiving is a strangely satisfying experience. Some keep journals or diaries, and some have tried poetry ("poetry instead of tears," as one caregiver put it). You can do such writing at odd moments, when your loved one is asleep or watching an old movie, or when you cannot sleep at night. In the process you will come to a deeper understanding of who you are and what you are going through.

One caregiver, Esther, who cared for her husband, Abe, for nearly ten years, wrote essays and poems in her diary during the entire course of her active caregiving as well as after her husband's death. With her permission, and that of her publisher, I will provide some insights from her writing here and elsewhere in this book.

From *Dear Alzheimer's: A Caregiver's Diary and Poems*, Esther Altshul Helfgott (Yakima, Washington: Cave Moon Press, 2013):

The Almost Widow

I have read in a number of places that a woman married to a man with Alzheimer's disease is living a widow's life. In the two-and-a-half years since my husband's diagnosis, I have not felt a sense of widowhood, but last night at a social function I did feel I am living the life of an almost widow. Here at the table were a handful of couples, each, while engaged with everyone else in the group, as I was, were also happily engaged with each other.

Now . . . my husband's initiative is gone, as is his possibility for arranging and participating in a social life . . . I arrange his day, and another caregiver is there when I am not. I help him with personal care, meals and all activities. His freedom is pretty much gone. Often I feel that mine is, too. Still, we manage, with pleasant moments weaving in and out of those that exhaust us both.

By the time I realized that I had settled into the role of spousal caregiver, my role had changed to include the experience of mourning the relationship that . . . had been. Getting out as an almost widow, whether to a . . . concert or an art exhibit, was not going to be as easy as buying a ticket or calling some friends. I was taking the Alzheimer's relationship with me, leaving at least three quarters of myself at home with my husband's silent gaze.

I have been attending support groups for Alzheimer's caregivers . . . and participating in the online Alzheimer's community. Both are helpful, but in each a component has been missing for me: discussion of grief and a focus on mourning before an actual death. And with Alzheimer's death is a daily occurrence.

Not everyone needs support groups, but for me they work toward helping me . . . understand the grief process. When I leave my home, grief is my escort. . . . An almost widow is not a widow. The relationship that used to be has taken a different form, but wherever I go, Abe and his illness are with me.

Secondary Caregivers

There are other members of your family who have an interest in the well-being of your loved one: your children, a brother or sister, an in-law, or other "interested parties." These individuals may at times tell you that you should be doing something else for your loved one than what you are doing. Your role as the primary caregiver of your loved one will always be to listen, and to consider whatever advice is given, but *you* need to be the one to decide whether to heed that advice or not. One of the ways of dealing with such advice is to ask the person giving you advice to participate in the caregiving process, perhaps to spell you for an afternoon so that you can attend to some other things.

Conflicts with others over the care of your patient can get quite emotional. Let us say your daughter thinks that you should admit your spouse to a nursing home, but you strongly disagree. There are no simple answers to this situation. Discuss the issue with the doctor or with members of your caregiver group, and bring the opinion of these other "experts" to bear on the issue. As I have said, listen always. Consider always as well, but comply only when the advice really makes sense to you, and/or to the doctor, or the group of peers in your support group.

Above All, Take Great Care of Yourself

It can be difficult to accomplish, but it is absolutely essential that you take excellent care of yourself during your loved one's illness. You need to continue to have "a life of your own" for your own sake as well as for the sake of your loved one. You cannot afford to neglect your own health care, grooming, leisure activities, rest and recreation, and so on. If you go "down the tubes," your loved one is sure to follow. So you need to make time for yourself, in this stage of the disease and, even more importantly, later.

Become Your Own Best Friend

As a caregiver a lot will be expected of you, while what is given to you may well shrink a bit. You may have less time for your friends, your church, or community group. You may be less able to attend parties, do things on impulse, or "just for the fun of it." That is why I would like to advise you to "become your own best friend." This may involve growing a somewhat thicker skin and being more ready to forgive yourself when you are less than perfect, even as you become more forgiving of interruptions and irritations inadvertently caused by your loved one. For other ideas about how to care for yourself, skip ahead to Chapters 17 through 20.

Chapter Summary

1. Early on in the process, you are still only a "caregiver in waiting."

2. Around this time, you should begin working with an elder-law attorney to obtain a durable family power-of-attorney and become a healthcare surrogate. The attorney can also assist with your loved one's last will and testament.

3. Sometimes a patient completely denies any impairment. This situation can be very difficult for caregivers and families.

4. Deciding whether your loved one needs to be told that he or she has Alzheimer's disease requires thoughtful consideration.

5. Caregiving is a job: it requires a plan and a schedule—one that includes at least one fun activity each day for you and your loved one.

6. As soon as possible, join a support group. The guidance and encouragement you gain will be invaluable, and you can help others after you learn your way.

7. Take great care of yourself, physically and emotionally. Writing about your experiences can be a creative outlet for your feelings and help you learn more about yourself during this challenging time.

Chapter 14

The Middle Stages: Patience and Humor

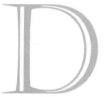URING the middle stages of Alzheimer's disease, almost all patients benefit most from receiving care in their own homes. This is true for a number of reasons. First, your loved one does not need to learn a new environment—he or she at least starts out knowing where everything is. His or her home, no matter how humble, contains more comforts and conveniences than any facility could, no matter how expensive, because these comforts are those that are familiar to the patient. In addition, no additional costs are involved.

Increasingly, too, it will become important that the caregiver maintain for the patient a stable, friendly, calm, and reassuring environment, free of chaos. Excessive noise and very bright lights are to be avoided, and furniture should stay in one place as much as possible. A stable, predictable routine of activities and meals is also essential. These steps help to avoid confusion, anxiety, irritability, or agitation in the patient, and they allow the caregiver to stay calmer and more relaxed. This is important because caregiving becomes even more demanding at this stage of the disease. In fact, before you become overwhelmed by the rising demands on your skills, your patience, and your creativity, I would like you to think about one other opportunity that you and your loved one have to contribute to a better understanding of Alzheimer's disease.

Should You Arrange for a Brain Autopsy?

The suggestion that a patient should arrange for a brain autopsy at the end of his or her Alzheimer's disease is a delicate matter, and views on this issue vary by personal, religious, and cultural background. But you should know that arranging for an eventual brain autopsy on your loved one is another opportunity for contributing to research on Alzheimer's disease. In order to do so, the principal caregiver, after consultation with other family members, must apply to and be accepted by a brain bank in your geographic area. The term *brain bank* reflects just how valuable this precious gift is for scientists, who are dependent on tissue samples to conduct high-quality studies of Alzheimer's disease. Most memory disorder clinics have a brain bank coordinator associated with their facility, and if you think your loved one would be interested, now is the time to contact that coordinator to learn more. If you and your patient decide to go ahead with an eventual donation, you will receive, in addition to the gratitude of the research community for this amazing contribution, a detailed report of the findings of the brain autopsy.

Caregiving Becomes More Challenging

It will come as no surprise to those of you helping someone in the middle stages of Alzheimer's disease that caregiving becomes tougher as the disease progresses. Many more areas of the patient's functioning are now affected. Virtually all of the areas we have been considering—memory, activities of daily living, hygiene and toileting, and mood and behavioral problems—are affected.

Coping with Worsening Memory Problems

Patients may now experience not only short-term memory impairments but long-term memory loss as well. Just in case it is not clear what is meant by long-term memory, let me offer a couple of illustrations. Patients with short-term memory problems may forget appointments, be unable to remember what or when they had breakfast, lose track of the date, or forget who has visited them over the past few days. People with long-term memory problems are unable to recall details of events from earlier in their lives. For instance when asked what their job had been, they might reply that they "had a very good job," or that they "worked very hard," rather than being able to name their specific position or occupation. When asked where they went to college, they might reply that they went to college "up North," or that they went to "a very good college." For the caregiver the same advice applies as before: don't try to "jog" the patient's memory. Don't say, "Oh, you must remember where you went to college!" If the patient doesn't know what date it is, don't insist that he or she try to remember or even point out the lapse. In the patient's reality, that information is no longer there, and, in fact, in the patient's view *it doesn't matter.*

As both short-term (recent) and long-term (remote) memory become increasingly impaired, the caregiver will need to fill in forgotten details where needed, or gloss over the issue of failed memory. Don't say "You know that" or "I already told you three times." Nothing is to be gained by dwelling on the fact that the patient cannot remember the information. Nor is there any benefit in correcting the patient when he or she "remembers" something that the caregiver knows is not true. When meeting people, the caregiver should help the patient by clearly identifying the person being greeted, rather than assuming that the patient will remember independently.

Dealing with Changes in Self-Care

Patients in the middle stages of Alzheimer's disease will now require more assistance with everyday activities: they may not be able to use the TV remote, or set the thermostat properly, or use a microwave oven, or perform other somewhat complex tasks.

Driving

When should an Alzheimer's patient stop driving? This is a very important question. In our society our sense of independence is very much connected to being able to come and go as we please. In Alzheimer's disease, judgment and reaction speed may become impaired well before the straightforward skills of operating an automobile decline. For this reason, patients with Alzheimer's disease should be persuaded fairly early on in the disease to trade off their own driving for being driven by their caregiver or by someone else. The risks of incurring an accident that may harm the patient or another person on the road, as well as the risk of financial loss due to an accident, are great indeed. When the patient with Alzheimer's disease cannot be persuaded to give up driving voluntarily, the patient's doctor should recommend to the patient and to the Bureau of Motor Vehicles that the person not drive any more. If need be, you as a caregiver may want to disable the patient's automobile, openly or surreptitiously, so that the Alzheimer's patient will no longer be able to drive.

Coping with Hygiene and Toileting Problems

At this point in the course of his or her disease, your patient may start to need much more prompting and supervision with his or her grooming and dressing. Always give only simple instructions, one step at a time, instead of stringing a whole series of instructions together. For instance, you can say: "Now put the toothpaste on your toothbrush." Then wait for that action to be accomplished before going on to the next step. To help your loved one get to the bathroom on time, it will be best to establish a routine of taking him or her to the toilet approximately every two hours, "whether you need it or not," in order to avoid embarrassing incontinence. Some patients begin to urinate in inappropriate places, such as in a wastebasket—if so, even closer supervision will be required. This may also be the time to introduce adult diapers to your patient to avoid embarrassing accidents. Some patients may resist this initially, but a calm and factual approach will usually lead to acceptance—though as one caregiver noted, after her mother easily accepted the need for adult diapers, there was another surprise:

My mother had always washed out her under-
wear at night and unfortunately when she went
into Depends, she'd try to wash those too. Need-
less to say, I dealt with clogged sinks a lot.

Often at this point in their illness, patients become
reluctant to take a bath or a shower. It is not just a matter of forgetting to wash; they may be frightened by
having water hit them suddenly in an enclosed space,
especially if the temperature of the water has not been
tested beforehand. Sometimes it may be possible to offer
a leisurely "spa" activity with the caregiver as a way of
coaxing the patient into the bath or shower.

Sex

The sexual behavior of patients with Alzheimer's
disease is likely to change, along with other changes in
their behavior, as the disease progresses. But there is no
single pattern of such changes. In some patients interest
in sex disappears, and while that may be regrettable, it
is part and parcel of the general loss of interest experienced by many patients. It is by no means the worst problem for the caregiver to deal with. More troublesome

may be two other types of changes in sexual behavior: an excessive preoccupation with sex and/or an excessively frequent demand for sex. Alternatively, the patient may be interested in having sex, but no longer remembers his or her own role in performing sexual acts. If this happens to you as a caregiver, seek advice from your own physician or your Alzheimer's patient's doctor. Other members in your support group will have faced similar issues as well, and they may have suggestions to offer to you regarding how to cope with the problem.

Sleep Apnea

Sleep apnea is a phenomenon that can occur in patients with and without Alzheimer's disease. A patient with sleep apnea will stop breathing while sleeping for a minute or so, and then breathe very deeply—even to the point of gasping—to restore the oxygen balance in his or her body. Sleep characterized by sleep apnea is not as refreshing as regular sleep, and may make memory function even worse. In non-Alzheimer's patients a mask providing positive pressure oxygen can remedy the situation. Unfortunately, such a mask is generally poorly tolerated by Alzheimer's patients. The use of medications like Provigil or Nuvigil may reduce the frequency and the severity of sleep apnea.

Weight Changes

In the early or middle stages of dementia, weight gain may become an issue, as the patient loses track of how much and how often he or she is eating, and in many cases becomes more sedentary. Weight gain can complicate caregiving as it may increase joint symptoms and make it harder to lift or move the patient. For these reasons, closer supervision of what foods are being served and eaten by the patient is indicated when he or she starts to gain weight.

When weight loss begins to occur in a patient with advanced Alzheimer's disease, in the absence of any other specific disease such as a gastrointestinal problem or cancer, it should be a warning sign that the end may be approaching. At this point the patient should be encouraged to eat frequent meals with high fat or calorie counts, such as ice cream, peanut butter, or fried foods that the patient can enjoy without worrying about cholesterol levels or diabetes. In general no heroic measures, such as tube feeding or intravenous feedings, are indicated for patients in the late stages of Alzheimer's disease.

Responding to More Severe Behavioral Problems

Behavior problems may also become more severe, requiring increasingly more creative responses on the part of the caregiver. Irritability and hostility may crop up with greater frequency. There may be lapses of tact, such as calling an overweight person fat to his or her face, or making inappropriate sexual overtures to acquaintances. Even though symptoms and deficits may be much more apparent now, a certain degree of denial will probably continue. Patients will tend to minimize or downplay their problems.

If you are like most caregivers, you will find the behavioral problems far more challenging than "mere" memory problems. Some patients, but by no means all of them, may now experience episodes of anxiety, depression, or agitation. Even worse, you may see irritability or outright hostility expressed toward you, the caregiver. If this should happen with your patient, you will need to acquire a number of new skills and techniques to stop the undesired activity. For example, when your patient first begins to express hostility toward you, you will want to take immediate and strong countermeasures. First of all, protect yourself at all costs, and in any way you can—even if you need to call for help from a neighbor or the police. Being hurt or injured by the person you are caring for is not part of your agreement to be a caregiver. Second, and amazingly, barking back at the patient in the manner of a drill sergeant often can abort an angry attack. You can even threaten to stop being the person's caregiver. One caregiver said to her angry husband: "If you ever do this again, I am going to send you to a nursing home." The patient stopped attacking her, and she never had to say it again.

Other techniques may include distracting or redirecting the patient. In my experience, redirecting is more effective than distracting. Redirecting means inviting the patient to do an entirely different activity: "Let's go for a walk," or "Let's go to McDonald's," or some other suggestion that might be appealing to the patient.

Also during this stage, hallucinations and/or delusions may occur for the first time. Hallucinations and delusions may be of two types, each of which has very different implications and requires a different type of response. The first type consists of images, voices, or beliefs that are what I call innocent distortions of reality. These hallucinations or delusions tend to "re-animate" the world of the patient with interesting but harmless visions, voices, or beliefs. One example of this might be a patient who complains that a cow is regularly coming into the living room. The patient sees the cow but others do not. The patient, however, is not afraid of the cow and is not threatened by the fact that there is a cow in his living room. For the innocent hallucination you have two choices: you can either go along with the hallucination without contradicting the patient, or you can become creative, as one caregiver did whose husband saw the cow in his living room. She agreed with him that there was a cow, and said to her husband, "Let's open the door and push the cow out of the room." She opened the door, pretended to push the cow out of the living room, and her husband was satisfied. The vision of the cow never returned.

Dangerous hallucinations and delusions, however, must be handled in quite a different way. Dangerous hallucinations or delusions are those in which the false perception or false belief places either the patient or the caregiver into imminent danger. An example might be when the patient hears voices telling him to kill the caregiver, or when he believes that his caregiver has poisoned him. Here the patient's doctor or an emergency room physician needs to be involved in order either to treat the patient with a major tranquilizer or possibly to hospitalize the patient in a secure psychiatric ward.

Keep on Keeping On

Some of the general caregiving strategies outlined in earlier chapters should continue during this stage of the disease as well. For example, you still have to be *so* gentle, and you still need to engage the patient in at least one pleasurable activity every day, although the nature of that activity may have to change according to the patient's response.

Overall, caregivers can expect to spend many more hours each day and each week doing something for or with the patient. Increasingly, the caregiver will find it necessary to share part of the burden of care with someone else, or to "outsource" some of the caregiving, by using outside resources such as daycare, respite care, and/or an assistant caregiver.

On Maintaining a Sense of Humor

Being able to respond to challenging circumstances with a sense of humor is a wonderful ability for anyone to have, and it is particularly useful to caregivers looking after an Alzheimer's patient. That does not mean that you are laughing *at* the patient or the behavior, but that you can and do see the funny aspects of any occurrence. One caregiver wrote down the following story for me about an event with her mother. She titled the story "A Walk on the Beach":

My mom has Alzheimer's disease. I try to do things with Mom. We have a place by the beach, and I asked if she wanted to go.

"Great," she said, "let's go."

We had a nice drive to the beach. We went up to our condominium and I asked her if she wanted to go for a walk on the beach.

"Yep," she said, "let's go."

I unpacked my swim suit and hers. We both have one-piece bathing suits, both of them blue with some other colors mixed in. I went into the bathroom to change and handed her her bathing suit to put on.

When I came out I saw that something looked funny. She turned around and I realized that she had put her bathing suit on front to back!

"Mom," I started to yell at her, "you've got your bathing suit on backwards!"

But I quickly realized that yelling at her was not going to be helpful. So I changed course. I took her over to the mirror, but she still didn't quite understand. She tried to hide her breasts behind the slim back straps, but it didn't quite work. So I helped her put on her bathing suit the right way. We both had a good laugh then and went out for a nice walk on the beach, as though nothing had happened. Well, I guess nothing had happened.

By making a lighthearted moment out of the occasion, the caregiver easily diffused the situation instead of treating it as a disaster. By writing down this story, too, the caregiver had a chance to reflect on a potentially awkward scenario and appreciate how she was still able to share a laugh and a connection with her mother.

Coping with a Loss of Social Inhibitions

When your loved one's social graces and inhibitions begin to deteriorate, and he or she begins to, say, make inappropriate remarks, or eat a meal with his or her fingers, other people may have strong reactions. To help ease their concerns, and to offer an explanation, you may want to have cards printed up that you can give to onlookers, restaurant servers, or even strangers, with this message: "Please excuse my loved one's behavior. He suffers from a memory disorder (Alzheimer's disease)." These cards can then be subtly slipped to the onlookers so that they can understand what is happening.

When Your Loved One Doesn't Recognize You

One of the most poignant events that can occur in the middle stages of Alzheimer's disease is the moment that the patient fails to recognize the caregiver, thinking instead that he or she is a total stranger, or is another member of the patient's family. Many caregivers are devastated when this happens. After all that they are doing and have done for their patient, how could such a thing happen? Well, it can and does happen to many devoted caregivers during the caregiving process, and being prepared can help make this moment less upsetting if it happens to you. You might try having in mind a couple of stories about some particularly meaningful moment in your relationship that only you could know. Retell the event to the patient, saying that you are the one that he or she surely remembers from that meaningful event. The patient may have an "aha!" moment and recognize you again, or you may need to let time pass and wait for another time when he or she will recognize you for who you are. Do not be dismayed if this happens. This is not your failure, and it is the disease speaking, not your loved one.

Seizures

A small proportion of patients with Alzheimer's disease may experience seizures solely as a result of the advancing Alzheimer's disease. If someone has seizures, a medical workup for other causes, such as tumors or strokes, should be carried out. But if no other causes are found, the patient should be treated with anti-seizure medications such as the drug Dilantin or a similar drug prescribed to minimize the risk that the seizures will recur.

Variations on a Theme

There are so many more challenges that can develop in the months and years of your caregiving experience that I cannot predict all of them for you. Keep an open mind, and try to understand what might be happening in the mind of your loved one when something unforeseen happens. "Let not your heart be troubled, neither let it be afraid," as the Bible says. And if you do develop some new technique for coping with unforeseen problems, be sure to share your wisdom with other caregivers. You can save them some trouble, and they will be grateful to you.

CHAPTER SUMMARY

1. The best place for an Alzheimer's patient to receive care during the middle stages of the disease is in his or her own home.

2. Before becoming overwhelmed by growing caregiver demands, decide with the patient's family whether there should be an eventual brain autopsy.

3. Caregiving will become much more difficult as the disease progresses, but you can also learn strategies to cope with your loved one's deteriorating abilities and the many changes that occur.

4. Keep your sense of humor; it will help you get through some of the tough times!

Chapter 15

The Late Stages:
Even More Challenging

I N THE later stages of Alzheimer's disease more and more abilities disappear, and the behavioral problems become much worse. The task of being a caregiver becomes much more challenging, in many ways. By this point in your loved one's care, you will need all the help you can get.

This may be a good time to reiterate the importance of continuing to give patients their anti-dementia medications. Even though your patient's behavior will not improve from taking these medications, be assured that they *are still working.* Discontinuing them would result in a much faster decline and worse behavioral problems. This has been demonstrated time and time again, and neither you nor your patient should have to go through such a disheartening experience. Yes, these medications may be expensive, but they continue to work to minimize symptoms. Research is currently under way to find medications that will not only hold back the disease, but will actually stop it from progressing.

Struggling to Communicate and Remember

At this point in your loved one's disease, his or her memory problems will have become much worse; both recent events and long-ago happenings will be more difficult to recall. Things you have just said to your loved one will not always be remembered, and you may have to repeat them time and again. The meaning of words will also begin to disappear. Not only will your patient not be able to understand exactly what you have said, but he or she will also not be able to find words to convey meaning. Patients at this stage may know exactly what they want to say, but will not be able to produce the word they are looking for. For example, they may point to a watch or a clock, but not be able to say the words "watch" or "clock."

Because verbal communications in this phase of the disease will have become quite limited, "yes" and "no" may be the only words patients can form regularly, and they may develop a kind of shorthand to express themselves. For instance, one patient used the single word "McDonald's" to indicate that he wanted to be taken to McDonald's for a hamburger. You will have to learn to guess or interpret what your loved one is trying to tell you. Just supply the missing word if you can guess it so the conversation can continue. Nothing is gained by insisting that your struggling loved one try to come up with the missing word—your goal should be to limit everyone's frustration and be as responsive and helpful as possible.

There will now almost certainly be times when your loved one does not recognize you—he or she may mistake you for someone else or for a stranger, and in fact even become frightened of you. This is really tough when someone you have lived with and loved for fifty years no longer knows who you are. Even more troublesome, the person you are caring for may at times no longer even recognize him- or herself. When looking in the mirror patients at this stage may ask: "What is that old man (or old woman) doing in my bathroom?" Some caregivers respond to this challenging situation by covering the mirrors around the house with towels until this phase of the disease passes.

Hallucinations and Delusions

As in the middle stages of the disease, there may be hallucinations and delusions. Hallucinations occur when someone suffering from Alzheimer's disease sees or hears something or someone whom you yourself cannot see or hear. Most of the time, these sensations are relatively benign and do not disturb the patient, although they may be upsetting to you. One of my patients, for example, used to see children coming into his living room, and his interpretation was that they were coming into this room because it was the only room in the house that was air-conditioned. At other times, patients may become severely frightened in response to these hallucinations, feeling they are in danger, or that they are being attacked. When this occurs, you will need to consult with the treating physician to see if additional medication or a tranquilizer may be indicated to help the patient get past this stage.

Delusions can be even more troublesome. One patient of mine regularly accused her caregiver husband of stealing her clothes from her closet. She would become very angry, go to complain about her husband to the neighbors, or sometimes even call the police. This caregiver husband was one of the most caring, loving, gentle persons you could imagine, but when his wife could not find something that she had misplaced, the accusations began. This situation required her doctor to prescribe increasing doses of a powerful tranquilizer. After several increases in the dose of the medication, the delusions disappeared, and she once again began to sing the praises of her husband, whom she described as "the best caregiver ever."

Depression, Apathy, and Anhedonia

Depression, apathy, and anhedonia (the word means "inability to experience pleasure") often occur in the later stages of Alzheimer's disease. Spontaneous activities will grind to a halt; the patient will not eat, get dressed, or participate in any activities. Trying to distract the patient or offering tender loving care may help, but sometimes additional medication will be needed. Interestingly, antidepressant medications are just as effective in dementia patients as they are in other patients. For apathy, too, doctors have tried to help by prescribing stimulant drugs such as those used in attention deficit/hyperactivity disorder (ADHD)—for example, Ritalin. The response to such medications varies widely, ranging from a real awakening of interest and emotion to little effect at all. Your loved one's physician can give you guidance on whether this might be a good approach to try with your patient. If your loved one is experiencing depression or apathy, be sure to bring this to the doctor's attention. Indeed, at this stage of the disease you will want to be in frequent contact with your patient's doctor, as well as in close touch with members of your support group who may have developed some skill or technique for dealing with one of the many behavioral problems that can occur.

Pervasive Negativism

Late in this disease there sometimes appears a pattern of behavior that is truly baffling and frustrating: the patient will say "no" to everything you propose, and no amount of explaining or reasoning will help. It may seem that the person is severely depressed and is unwilling or unable to give any positive responses. Sometimes it goes away after a period of time. You might be able to hasten its disappearance by offering tender love and affection, as well as verbal reassurances. A trial of antidepressant medication may also be indicated—ask your doctor for advice. Perhaps someone in your support group will come up with an answer to why this occurs. If you come across an answer, please let me know. My best guess is that pervasive negativism is an existential expression of the deep and utter frustration that someone must feel about having been afflicted with Alzheimer's disease.

Sleep Disturbances

Sleep disturbances may also occur and can even involve a complete reversal of the day-night cycle. This is a very troublesome development because if your patient cannot sleep, you are not going to be able to sleep either—a situation that will very quickly run you down physically and emotionally. If this happens, you may need to get help from friends or relatives to care for the patient for a few hours while you get some sleep. Exercise or other physical activities during the day may help your patient sleep more regularly, but sleep-inducing medication may also be needed, at least temporarily. This strategy is not without risk, since sleeping medications can further impair the patient's memory function and lead to daytime drowsiness as well as a more unsteady gait (and so an increased risk of falls). For a patient with Alzheimer's disease, a hip fracture or similar mishap can be devastating. Rehabilitation from such injuries is very difficult in a patient with Alzheimer's disease, and falls should be prevented by any means possible.

Toileting, Incontinence, and Adult Diapers

As the disease progresses, your patient will become less and less aware of when he or she needs to go to the bathroom. While in the middle stages you were probably able to avoid episodes of incontinence by taking your loved one to the bathroom every couple of hours, at this stage of the disease you will need to ease your patient into using adult disposable diapers. Many patients will resist this idea at first, and will initially refuse to wear such garments, either at night or in the daytime. But as the experience of wetting or soiling themselves becomes more frequent, and the cleanup process becomes more burdensome and unpleasant, most patients eventually accept having to wear such garments. While this lightens the burden on the caregiver somewhat, there is still the huge task of keeping the patient clean and dry at all times. Some caregivers, of course, will have had experience with diapering infants, and are therefore somewhat prepared. But providing incontinence care for adults is more complex. Accordingly I recommend that all caregivers become trained in incontinence care.

Training in Incontinence Care

Providing incontinence care requires the appropriate attitudes, approaches, and equipment so that changes can be accomplished in a matter-of-fact way, without embarrassment to patient or caregiver. The care needs to be provided calmly and efficiently, without causing an emotional disturbance every time it is undertaken. Perhaps your support group can arrange for a special training session on incontinence care given by a public health nurse or a nurse from a long-term care facility who has extensive experience in this area. Without such training, the onset of incontinence and misadventures in providing such care can lead to unnecessarily early admission to a residential care facility, or cause caregivers to give up. An interesting case history, which the daughter of an Alzheimer's patient crafted into a story she called "Afternoon Surprise," may illustrate the point:

> My mother has Alzheimer's disease, poor thing. She was diagnosed about a year ago after she got lost driving to the beauty parlor. She had only been going there once a week for the last three years, or as long as she had lived with John [a widower with whom the mother had an intimate relationship]. But that is another story. I took her to my own doctor and told him I was concerned about her memory, and that she had gotten lost the other day. The doctor asked her the date and gave her three words to remember, and she couldn't do either one. So he sent her to have an MRI done, and afterwards told me and her that she had "a memory problem." He didn't use the "A" word with her, but I knew. He told her he was going to put her on some medicine, Aricept, that would help her memory, to which she said "okay." That was a year ago.
>
> Today I came to pick her up to go grocery shopping, which she likes to do with me. Boy, did I get a surprise! As I drove up to John's house, I saw she was sitting on the front porch. In front of her were six suitcases all lined up: her two carry-on bags that she used to take on trips with her; an old cardboard suitcase that was

beginning to come apart; and three other cases that were more or less just moving boxes with string wrapped around them.

"What's up, Mom?" I said.

"I guess John doesn't want me anymore."

Just then John came out the front door, looking down, not looking me in the eye. I said: "What's up, John?" And he said, "Joanne, you're going to have to take your mom home with you. I just can't take it anymore. I'm sorry."

They had lived together for three years. He really seemed to care about her. He used to go to the doctor with her, and ask him questions about what he was supposed to do.

The doctor had told me: "When she becomes incontinent, he may not be able to handle it anymore." So I guess I had been warned. I put my arms around Mom, and she hers around me, and we both had a good cry. Then I loaded four of the suitcases in the back of my station wagon, and put the two carry-on bags on the back seat. Then we both got in my car and drove off.

This story illustrates how difficult it may be for a caregiver to provide incontinence care, and perhaps especially, in our culture, for a man to give such care to a woman. In this situation, where the "significant other" had known the patient for only a short period of time, he was unable to cope with this task in an ongoing way. Clearly, there was pain on both sides, and the daughter did what she had to do. She stepped in to fill the void.

Sudden Behavioral Changes May Signal New Problems

When patients experience sudden behavioral changes, such as agitation or frantic pacing, caregivers need to be alert to the possibility that the patient is experiencing pain or another new medical problem. Since patients at this stage have major difficulties expressing themselves verbally, they can resort to this alternate method of signaling that "something is wrong." The "something" could be anything from a severe toothache to infection somewhere in the body, or even a heart attack. You should check your loved one's vital signs (pulse, blood pressure, body temperature), and if these don't reveal anything about the cause of the changed behavior, arrange for a general medical examination by a physician to be done as soon as possible. If an appointment cannot be arranged with the patient's regular doctor, a visit to an emergency clinic or a neighborhood walk-in clinic may help you figure out what may be wrong.

Screaming: A Need to Be Heard?

When patients at home or in a care facility suddenly begin to scream, it is not only disruptive and distracting; it may also mean that they are trying to communicate something very important about themselves. They quite possibly are feeling frightened, lost, or desperate in response to their condition. If your loved one starts screaming all of a sudden, know that there is no point in asking "What's wrong?" You already know that he or she can no longer express feelings in words. Instead focus on providing tender loving care, whether by putting an arm around your patient, giving hugs, smiling, saying "there, there, there" repeatedly, or even offering ice cream or chocolate, which sometimes seems to help abate screaming episodes. Screaming in a care facility might also indicate that your patient is having too little interaction with staff and other residents. It sometimes takes a little detective work for a caregiver to figure out what is wrong. Until then, give lots of love and attention—these remedies hardly ever have any unwanted side effects.

When Your Loved One Needs a Care Facility

As the burdens of caregiving increase, you will need to face what may be one of the most agonizing decisions you will ever make: when to place your loved one into a care facility especially designed for memory-impaired persons. As the person you are caring for becomes less and less able to cooperate with you, in terms of dressing and bathing, but especially in terms of getting to the bathroom on time, it will be best to consider finding a place where more than one person will be able to provide the needed care. This means admission to either an assisted living facility or a specialized memory care unit in a nursing home. But this is a task that you need to plan ahead for; you don't want to make such important decisions in haste. In fact, since this process is complex and loaded with lots of emotion on all sides, I will devote the entire next chapter to a full discussion of what is involved.

Hospice Care

There is one other type of care that you may wish to consider for your loved one in the late stages of Alzheimer's disease. When someone has reached the stage in medical care where full recovery is not possible, hospice care can be instituted. Hospice care provides end-of-life care that is devoted to making the patient comfortable. Those who are experiencing pain can be kept pain-free with a regimen of powerful medications, without concern about becoming addicted. Hospice care is perhaps most commonly used for patients dealing with the end stages of terminal cancer. But it can also be used for someone in the late stages of Alzheimer's disease, heart disease, chronic obstructive pulmonary disease, or any other terminal condition. Care is provided either in the patient's own home or in a homelike setting, but it can also be provided for someone in a nursing home. Psychological comfort and communication with family members and friends are emphasized. Importantly, hospice care is provided at no additional cost as a regular Medicare or Medicaid benefit.

Hospice services may include ongoing care by physicians, nurses, social workers, or mental health specialists. An important aspect of hospice care is that trained volunteers make up a significant proportion of the hospice personnel. Such volunteers can provide emotional support and companionship, run errands, or provide transportation.

CHAPTER SUMMARY

1. During the later stages of Alzheimer's disease, patients' memory problems are much worse, their verbal communications become quite limited, their behavioral problems become more prominent, and they struggle with toileting and incontinence.

2. Adult diapers become needed around this time. Be sure to become trained in incontinence care to help the process go more smoothly for both you and your loved one.

3. Be alert for sudden behavioral changes, which may indicate pain or a new medical problem. A patient's screaming may indicate a need to be heard.

4. Now is the time to plan ahead for the possibility that your loved one will need to be placed in a full-time care facility.

5. Hospice care may be an option for patients in the very last stages of Alzheimer's disease.

Chapter 16

The Hardest Decision You'll Ever Make

CAREGIVING is a very challenging activity and over the course of a patient's illness, caregivers face many difficult and often unexpected problems. That is why I recommend that caregivers get help as early as possible and continue to get help throughout the process, from caregiver support groups as well as health professionals, family members, and friends. But there is one decision that is more difficult to face than any other: placement of a loved one into a special care facility.

Do It for the Right Reason: Your Loved One's Care

Earlier on in this book I advised that, for most stages of Alzheimer's disease, the best place for patients to receive care is in their own home. But when your loved one has become extremely dependent, can no longer cooperate with you, or has developed unmanageable behaviors, a specially designed and specially staffed facility will be the best place for him or her to receive care. Why? Because generally no one person can deal with the increased care demands, which may include getting the patient in and out of bed, handling more frequent or complicated incontinence care, or coping with hostile and aggressive behavior.

Fortunately there are now a number of types of facilities that are able to provide excellent care for your loved one. These include Alzheimer's assisted living facilities and specialized memory care units in nursing homes. The critical component of these units is not the label "Alzheimer's care unit" or "memory-impaired unit" but whether the staff of such a unit is specially trained in caring for memory-impaired individuals. An Alzheimer's assisted living facility will be appropriate for individuals who can still handle basic self-care tasks such as eating, dressing, and getting in and out of bed. A memory-impaired unit in a nursing home will be appropriate for individuals who have come to need assistance in feeding, dressing, and toileting.

Prepare Early

Since placement in a care facility is a possibility, perhaps even a probability, for many Alzheimer's patients in the late stages of their disease, caregivers need to prepare for such an eventuality. When you begin to observe worsening dependency and/or increasingly unmanageable behaviors in your patient, you should begin to check out facilities available in your community. You should personally (but without the patient) visit several such facilities, meet with staff members, and talk to other caregivers who have patients staying there. I recommend that you make several visits at different times of the day to facilities you are interested in, paying special attention to the ratio of staff to patients at these differing times.

Don't Try to Make This Important Decision Alone

You should definitely seek the advice of your loved one's doctor at this time so that you can be assured that the decision is based on objective observations, not only on emotional factors. Consulting the doctor may also help to reduce any guilt feelings you might experience, or any guilt feelings that the patient or other family members may wish to induce in you. Talking with your caregiver support group about the particulars of your case may also provide emotional support for what is clearly a difficult decision, and the other caregivers may also be able to share their experiences with specific facilities in your community.

A New Stage of Caregiving

One husband, Harry, confided in me how he felt about admitting his wife, Mary, to a specialized memory care unit in a nursing home. Clearly devoted to continuing his loving connection with her no matter where she was, he said: "When she no longer knows that she and I belong together, then I'll be able to let her go." Harry continued to visit his wife in the nursing home every day until she finally passed away. This anecdote only reinforces the fact that with admission of your loved one to a special care facility, you will not be shut out from further caregiving. In fact, the contrary is true: a whole new phase of your caregiving career is beginning. You will want to supervise and assure yourself that the most appropriate care is indeed being provided, and if it is not, you will need to gently but firmly bring your concern to the attention of facility staff. You will also need to decide how often you will visit the facility, both initially and then over the longer term, as well as whether and how often you might want to take your loved one out of the facility, either for a meal or to return to visit the patient's former home. (The home-visit discussion is one that you will probably want to share with the facility staff, since taking your patient away from the facility might lead him or her to create a scene or outright refuse to return to the "new home.")

I also strongly recommend, in part to affirm that you are still a caregiver, that you continue to attend your caregiver support group. You may wish to continue with the same group that has supported you thus far, or you may wish to switch to a caregiver group operated by the care facility where your loved one is placed. A new group might be more focused on what both you and your patient are experiencing right now.

"But I Promised I Would Never Put Her in a Nursing Home"

Many times I have heard a caregiver utter this phrase, in complete agony, as he or she is considering the need to find a facility for ongoing care of a loved one, whether a wife, a husband, or a mother. While I would like to advise all caregivers not to make such promises to their loved ones, by the time they tell me it is often too late, and such promises have been made. Yet they also clearly made that promise to their loved one when he or she was an entirely different person. The caregiver is faced with the need to responsibly and lovingly make another choice now that the patient is himself or herself in a very different mental and physical state.

Keep in mind, too, that the image of a nursing home that you or your loved one may have in mind may be very outdated: nursing-care facilities today no longer have smelly hallways, minimal attention to the needs of the patients, and a staff untrained in dealing with memory-impaired patients. Today you will be able to find a nursing home that specializes in caring for memory-impaired persons in a homelike atmosphere, with a full range of activities geared to the abilities of its residents, and a kind, attentive staff that is willing and able to speak with you, the responsible caregiver, whenever you need to do so. You may need to visit several facilities to find the right one for your loved one, but you can do it. Be sure to ask members of your caregiver support group for names and ideas for where to start your search.

Even if you take care to make a loving choice for your patient, it is never easy to have to place a loved one into a facility. One caregiver described his agony at seeing his wife in the care facility, with her shrinking abilities, fading personality, and diminishing ability to recognize him, writing:

> Try to imagine [that] while you are out of town, lightning strikes your house and it burns to the ground. This is the home you've loved and lived in for decades. Your neighbor tells you the news and you come right back.
>
> You park out front and there is the location and the lot and the foundation, but the structure that made it a house is gone and it is just a smoldering bed of gray ashes. All the possessions, valuables, heirlooms, photos, memorabilia, and memories that made it home are gone too and lie in those ashes.
>
> Your emotions well up as you contemplate what you have lost. It's beyond your comprehension, you can't grasp it all at once, and you are left hanging. And it is all so clearly final.
>
> That's what it is like when I visit my wife, in the care facility where what remains of her

resides. The familiar foundation is there, but the intellect, the spirit, the emotion, the responses, that had made her a loving wife for so many years, are gone. And it is all so clearly final.

Placing a loved one in a special care facility is certainly an emotionally difficult task. It is not only a big transition for your loved one, but also the start of a new stage for you as a caregiver and person. It is important at this time that you ask for and accept help from family members and friends. Take this opportunity to begin to reduce some of the isolation you have been experiencing, reintegrate into your larger community, and even allow yourself some small indulgences that you have been denying yourself.

CHAPTER SUMMARY

1. The time will come when you will need to consider placing your loved one in a care facility, since this will almost certainly be the best place for your patient to receive care during the late stages of Alzheimer's disease.

2. Do not try to make the decision entirely alone about where and when to place your loved one in a care

facility. Doctors, friends and family members, and your caregiver support group are essential resources at this time, and can help you begin your search for good facilities in your area.

3. Placing your loved one in a care facility does not mean that you will be shut out from further caregiving. In fact the contrary is true: you will continue to be your patient's emotional and healthcare advocate, which is a demanding and essential job.

4. Even if earlier in your loved one's illness you promised never to put him or her in a care facility, at this late stage in the disease your patient has changed—he or she is no longer the same person who heard this promise, and now needs more comprehensive help. You should never feel guilty for making a loving, responsible choice about the care of your patient.

PART IV

TAKING CARE OF YOURSELF

Chapter 17

Caregivers Need Care, Too

ANY of the chapters so far have been devoted to the topic of what a patient needs from his or her caregiver. Now it is time to turn to your needs—the needs that you, the caregiver, have as an individual as well as in your caregiving role. Early on in my work with caregivers I was struck by the fact that for all that caregivers gave, they themselves had many unmet needs. In short, I realized that caregivers need care, too.

What kind of care do most caregivers need? To start with, information about the illness they are dealing with and its course; emotional support and recognition for the many contributions they are making; knowledge about community resources as well as legal and financial issues; and practical information for coping with a patient's troublesome behaviors. They also need to understand the nature of the caregiver role, and how to protect their own well-being and self-esteem.

Be Sure to Join a Caregiver Support Group

As I've mentioned elsewhere, one of the best things that a caregiver can do is to join an Alzheimer's caregiver support group. In a caregiver support group you will meet regularly with perhaps a dozen other caregivers with whom you can share and from whom you can learn any number of techniques that you can immediately apply for dealing with issues as they arise. The leader of such a group should have a deep understanding of Alzheimer's disease and the role of caregivers, as well as skills related to group counseling.

Most caregivers feel that participation in a support group not only nurtures them but also has a profound healing effect. As part of a well-functioning group, they will find that they can bring up any kind of question at all that is troubling them without fear of disapproval or fear of not being taken seriously. A caregiver group is a safe place in which to express anger (why us?), frustration, guilt, even issues related to one's sex lives. More often than not, any new problem that crops up for someone has already been dealt with by someone else. And even if that is not the case, members of the caregiver group will often work out a possible solution to that problem and any other number of ever-changing problems that one of their members is facing. Information about new opportunities, such as participation in a promising clinical study, will also spread like wildfire among the group. Often I have heard from caregivers who did not have the advantage of belonging to a caregiver group that they felt as if they were missing out on a vital lifeline.

To be sure, not all groups will meet the needs of everyone looking for a support group. One experienced caregiver advises that you try more than one group, both to learn some things from one group and some from another and to find the group that fits you best. Caregiver support groups are made up of all kinds of people: men and women, spouses and ex-spouses, sons and daughters, sons-in-law and daughters-in-law, each bringing a somewhat different point of view to the caregiver experience. As one participant wrote about Alzheimer's caregiver support groups:

I have attended numerous meetings of support groups for people caring for family members suffering from senile dementia of the Alzheimer type. During this time I have gradually become aware of an interesting feature. There is a substantial difference between those persons caring for a spouse and those caring for a parent. The two groups have significantly different views of the problems, the ways to cope with them, the outcomes they hope for and especially of their interactions with the patient. When more than one child is involved in a parent's care, the differences are even greater and more obvious.

I conclude that the basic reason for this is that when a couple marries they tend to grow closer to each other, while as children grow and mature they tend to grow apart from their parents. There is a rather stable period of decades from the time the children become independent until the parents succumb to old age. Then, a whole new relationship starts to develop as the child grows closer to the parent but now with the caregiving roles reversed. This new relationship is foreign to both parties and very difficult for each to understand and accept. Meanwhile, the spouses continue caring for each other as before, to the extent that each is still able.

This situation is entirely natural and normal. It is neither right nor wrong. It is simply a fact of life. Now that I have finally recognized it and brought it into focus, it has helped me to understand and evaluate the remarks and feelings of the other members of the support groups and has influenced the way I now respond to those members.

Learning to Share the Burden of Care

Despite what you may have believed at the outset, it is possible, no, it is *necessary,* to share the burden of care for someone with Alzheimer's disease. It is quite natural that you may want to do everything yourself, perhaps because you fear that no one else will be able to do as good a job of caring for your loved one as you can—and you are right. But there will be times when it will be wise for you to share parts or all of the job with someone else.

To illustrate that you are not alone in hesitating to delegate any part of the caregiving task to someone else, let me tell you about one such situation, the case of Manuel and Cathy:

Manuel was a successful businessman, community leader, and philanthropist. He and his wife, Cathy, were very close. They went everywhere together. At age seventy, Cathy began to repeat herself incessantly; she often misplaced her keys, lost her checkbook, and needed to be reminded about appointments she had. At first, Manuel tried to rationalize Cathy's forgetfulness and hide his concern about her from friends and family members. He didn't want to believe that she could possibly be developing Alzheimer's disease. As her symptoms continued to worsen, however, he became sufficiently concerned that he sought professional help. Cathy was evaluated, and doctors told Manuel that she did indeed have Alzheimer's disease. Cathy was quickly started on treatment. Early on, her doctor advised Manuel that he should consider seeking help with caring for his wife, but he insisted that he would be the only one to look after her. Both he and Cathy were very private people, and neither one wanted to accept the idea of a stranger coming into their home.

As Cathy became more and more impaired, and Manuel had to do more and more for her, he became increasingly depressed and tired, but he still refused to get any help with his caregiving duties. Cathy got up several times during the night, was agitated, and Manuel got very little sleep. Still, he insisted that he do everything for her, and that no one else could care for Cathy as well as he could. Then, within twenty-four hours, two things happened: Cathy got up in the middle of the night and fell in the bathroom, injuring her chest and her head; and Manuel himself injured his back trying to lift her from the bathroom floor. He finally called his daughter and allowed her to bring in live-in help for both of them. A few weeks later he confessed to Cathy's doctor, "I'm so relieved we have help now. I should have listened to your advice a lot sooner."

The take-home lesson from the story of Manuel and Cathy is to share the burden of care sooner rather than later. This is for your benefit as well as for the good of your loved one. If you can introduce additional help at a stage when your loved one can still form new relationships easily, it will ease the need to accept additional help later on in the course of the illness. It really does take a team of caregivers to provide all the help that is needed. Have no fear; you will always be the head of the team: but let others play a supporting role. Your life and that of your loved one will be richer for it. There will be less pain, less grief, less isolation. So allow yourself to be helped!

The Dangers of Not Accepting Help

If you think I have gone overboard in insisting that you seek and get help early on in your caregiver experience, let me tell you the stark reality of why I am so concerned. First of all, caregivers are not invulnerable. Without help they can become discouraged, depressed, or suffer burnout, and as a result they can begin to neglect their own care or the care of their patient. Some totally distressed caregivers can even become abusive to their loved ones when they feel at the end of their rope. You don't want to be among them. Caregiver assistance helps prevent such outcomes.

But there is yet another reason for careful planning and for assuring that someone else can provide some of the care needed: it is possible that you may die before your loved one. You may have an accident, develop an unforeseen medical problem, or fall victim to a natural or civil disaster. Planning ahead and sharing the burden of care will mean that your loved one will have a safety net in place just in case something happens to you.

The Benefits of Adult Daycare

As part of my advice to you as a caregiver to "share the burden of care," I recommend that you consider having your loved one participate in an adult daycare program for memory-impaired people. This option can be especially appropriate and beneficial during the long months and years when the patient is in the middle stages of the disease. (In the early stages of the disease the patient may resent going, perhaps because he or she sees it as demeaning, whereas in the very late stages he or she may not be physically or mentally able to participate.) Adult daycare programs offer many stimulating and fun activities, including socializing, reminiscing, dancing, simple exercises, listening to music or sing-alongs, or watching movies. The socialization with staff and with other patients that goes on in daycare programs is also of great benefit to the patients. And not unimportantly, adult daycare gives you, the caregiver, time for yourself for those hours each day that your loved one participates. Some programs are open as many as five times a week, or even on weekends. Use those times to attend to your own needs, go to the beauty parlor or the barbershop, play golf, go to the doctor, socialize with your friends, attend church, or just have fun. Give yourself permission to enjoy life and to do whatever will contribute to your own health and happiness during these hours. You will return to caregiving so much more refreshed and restored.

The cost of participating in daycare programs is generally low, because these programs are usually either supported by public funding, offer a sliding-scale fee system that takes into account your financial situation, or both. Adult daycare programs may be operated by memory disorder clinics, councils on aging, assisted living facilities, or even as freestanding not-for-profit operations.

Respite Care

While having your patient attend adult daycare will give you short periods of relief, certain events may crop up in your life that require a longer period of time away from caregiving: the wedding of an adult child or other relative, a graduation from college, a family reunion, or even an elective medical procedure. You might even just need a much deserved, honest-to-goodness vacation. For occasions like this, I recommend that you consider placing your patient into a *respite care program.* Respite care for a week or two, sometimes even up to three weeks, is provided by a number of enlightened assisted living facilities or nursing homes that operate special memory care units. Your loved one will receive excellent care there while you are away, and you both will look forward to being reunited when you return. Sometimes respite care stays can also serve as a preview of the kind of care your patient might receive at such a facility, since you may eventually have to consider placing your loved into such care. But I would keep this part of your purpose to yourself for now.

The cost of respite care programs also is generally affordable, and it may be supported by charitable organizations. The Alzheimer's Association conducts such programs in many communities, as do some nursing homes, in part as a marketing tool. The Veterans Administration also offers respite care to eligible veterans. Again, cost should not stand in the way of using this highly beneficial service.

Start a Caregiver Exchange

Another "invention" that I have seen some caregivers create is a caregiver exchange program. You trade off caregiving for your patient with another like-minded, loving caregiver, so that each of you in turn will take care of two patients who are compatible with one another while the other takes a much-needed break. Like these other options, caregiver exchanges are designed to benefit both participating caregivers and their patients.

Take Your Loved One on a Cruise

You may be surprised to learn that cruises for a few days (up to two weeks) are almost ideal ways of giving both you and your loved one a break. If a cruise sounds appealing, plan to take it during the early or middle stages of the disease, so that your loved one can still maneuver about and enjoy the sights and sounds, entertainment and activities, and meals under your supervision. Careful planning needs to go into any cruise vacation to assure that it will not be too demanding for either one of you, and if you're not sure if it will be too much, you can think about taking a relative or friend along to share the caregiving duties. But you may just find that the self-contained environment of a cruise offers a wonderful getaway for both you and your patient.

And don't forget to tell your caregiver support group about the experience when you return! I bet you will get a round of applause, and possibly a little bit of envy.

Recruit and Deputize an Assistant Caregiver

At any stage of the disease you can certainly find and train somebody else as a deputy caregiver. This could be a sibling who doesn't have time for caregiving all the time, a friend, someone from your church or other social group, or your spouse. You could also hire someone, if there is not someone in your circle who could provide the occasional caregiver break to you. Consider hiring a college student or a retired person who could use the extra money, or use your imagination or the combined imagination of your caregiver support group to come up with another likely candidate. Your loved one will surely come to enjoy the change of pace that comes with receiving care from someone else, even if he or she is not happy about it at first. I certainly have seen this strategy work very effectively in many cases, and in many different ways.

Like the other strategies I suggest in this book, this

way of sharing the burden of care is designed to maintain your physical and mental health, give you strength, and foster your capacity for caregiving.

CHAPTER SUMMARY

1. Most caregivers have many unmet needs, but taking care of yourself is a very important part of taking care of your loved one. Exhaustion and emotional burnout are very real dangers for caregivers of Alzheimer's patients. Don't let them happen to you!

2. Remember: an excellent way to gain perspective, new ideas, and friends who will appreciate the challenges you face is to join an Alzheimer's caregiver support group.

3. Don't forget to share the burden of care. Start sooner rather than later, and be sure to consider all the options, including adult daycare, respite care, caregiver exchanges, and recruiting an assistant caregiver.

4. Take a break, either by yourself or even with your loved one if you can find an easy, fun way to get away. Going on a cruise can be one such enjoyable option for caregivers and their patients during the earlier stages of Alzheimer's disease.

Chapter 18

Caregiver Support Groups

HEN I first became involved in conducting clinical studies back in 1968, when no medications for the treatment of Alzheimer's disease were yet available, I observed an interesting phenomenon: after caregivers brought their patients to the clinical studies and watched them disappear with one or another of the clinicians, they would get together with other caregivers and talk, talk, talk—or more precisely, share, share, share. It seemed that these caregivers felt a deep need to exchange information and to compare notes with other caregivers. And we began to respond to this need by establishing the first caregiver support groups, under the leadership of one of our team clinicians, a doctor, or a social worker or nurse.

Our initial groups were so successful that we soon began to promote the idea to other Alzheimer's study groups and to memory specialists in general. I am not claiming here that we were the only ones to come up with the concept of caregiver support groups, but it certainly spread like wildfire. It has now become an established practice in studies and clinical practices nearly everywhere, including long-term care facilities, special memory-disorder programs in nursing homes, and assisted living facilities. Some are operated by churches, and some by entrepreneurs who do nothing but run such groups, but the ubiquity of these groups confirms that they are a valuable resource for caregivers. When I think of how important they are, I remember a particularly memorable occasion in a recent caregiver group:

> Jill, a broadcaster for a local television station, came to the support group, looking not her usual self-possessed and confident self but upset and seemingly near tears. Of course members of the group and the group leader noticed this, and shortly after greeting everybody, they asked her what had transpired. She replied that her father who was in the late

stages of Alzheimer's had sat her down recently and told her, seemingly out of the blue: "Jill, I don't love you anymore." As Jill tried to tell her story, she dissolved in tears.

The group responded with both vocal and silent expressions of sympathy. The two group members sitting closest to her got up and put their arms around her. One of the members said, "Well, we still love you," but Jill continued to cry. At this point the leader of the group asked the group how they would have responded, or how Jill could have responded. One of them said, "That wasn't your dad talking; that was the disease talking." Others responded by saying they understood how she felt, given the enormous amount of care she was providing for her father.

Then the leader returned to the question of how Jill should have responded. One of the more experienced members of the group said, "You should have said 'But I still love you, Dad.'" Another member said that she would just look at the situation clinically, objectively, and not personally. After all, this expression was indeed a result of the father's disease. Easier said than done! But Jill gradually calmed down, wiped her tears from her face, and thanked the group for their understanding.

This is but one illustration of how time and again group members support one another and come up with creative solutions for some of the problems raised in the group.

The Genius of Caregiver Support Groups

The genius of caregiver groups is that they are inclusive communities into which members are invited at a very vulnerable time in their lives. For caregivers, becoming part of a new community at a time when they are really stressed, and to a significant degree isolated from other communities such as their church or their neighborhood groups, is a truly welcome relief. These groups vividly demonstrate to their members that they are not alone in their situation, and that others may have developed techniques and skills that they too can learn.

But it is not just a matter of learning needed skills. Equally important, or even more so, is the fact that this will be a group of people who will not be shocked by anything that is happening in your caregiver experience. They have been there before you and are there with you now. You can feel comfortable baring your soul, because they will understand. Before long, you will come to think of your caregiver group as family.

Caregiver Support Groups Can Vary Widely

Caregiver groups come in all shapes and sizes. Most often, groups have between seven and twenty-five members. With too few members, the group does not have enough variety and experience. With too many members, some members cannot be heard from at each session. Groups meet from once a week to once a month. Most groups are led by a health professional such as a nurse, social worker, physician, psychologist, or group facilitator. Large groups sometimes have co-leaders, with one professional and one lay leader. Group sessions last from one to two hours. Some groups are made up primarily of spousal caregivers, others attract mostly adult children—any mix of caregiver types is possible.

It's Okay to Try One or More Groups

New members can join at any time. Group members may leave, too, often either because their caregiving career has ended, they move away, or they simply want to try another support group with a different leader or a different composition of caregivers. That is, caregiver groups are quite flexible. They are there to serve caregivers. And while the participants spend a lot of their time learning how they can best serve their loved one, the primary focus in the support group is always the well-being of the caregivers themselves. As the flight attendants tell passengers on airplanes: "Put the oxygen mask on yourself first, before trying to help the person next to you." Experienced caregivers know well that if they do not take care of themselves first, they will not have the strength they need to give good care to others.

Chapter Summary

1. Caregiver support groups grew out of a natural desire to share helpful ideas and to seek advice and friendship with others during a challenging time.

2. The genius of caregiver groups is that everyone in the group can relate in some way to your experience, so you can bare your soul without feeling embarrassed or guilty.

3. Caregiver support groups can vary widely—don't feel shy about trying out different groups until you find one that feels right to you.

Chapter 19

When Your Loved One Dies

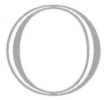NE insightful person describing the experience of caring for an Alzheimer's patient called it "the long good-bye." Over the months and years that you have seen your loved one lose characteristics and abilities that you once cherished, you have indeed in many ways been letting go and saying good-bye to him or her right along. Yet the finality of death is still something for which none of us is completely prepared. When the time comes for your loved one, you will experience a new kind of loss, a new kind of grief. There will be no one to visit, no one's hand to hold, and no one's brow to stroke. The loss will be devastating, even if you have been losing your loved one for years.

Grief—and Some Relief

If you are like most people, it is likely that, along with your grief, you will also feel a certain amount of relief that your loved one is now at peace, and that your task as a caregiver has come to an end. That is as it should be. Some people feel ashamed of these feelings, but this relief is entirely normal, and nothing to feel guilty about. Instead you can be proud for all that you have done, knowing that you made a positive difference in the life of your loved one at a time when he or she most needed it. You have been a good and faithful servant, and it is now time for this chapter of your life to end, to close the book on caregiving. It is now time to celebrate the life that has been laid to rest, remember fondly the affection and the commitment between you and your loved one, and appreciate the special bond you shared.

Of course, life goes on, even when it feels like it can't or shouldn't. You will be occupied with funeral arrangements, obituaries, memorial services, death certificates, and visitors, all of which are important, but they will still feel like nothing compared to the relationship you once had. It will be a time of remembering and a time of grieving. But first there is one decision you may need to make before all the others: whether to have a brain autopsy conducted on your loved one.

Considering a Brain Autopsy

As I mentioned earlier, there are very good reasons for having an autopsy performed at the time your loved one dies: (1) to confirm the diagnosis, and (2) to contribute to research on Alzheimer's disease. In general it is necessary to have the brain collected for examination as quickly as possible, usually within two to four hours after death. This can be done through whoever will be handling funeral arrangements, and it will not disturb the physical appearance of your loved one. If you do proceed, you will be told whether the physical hallmarks of Alzheimer's disease were in fact present in the brain of your loved one. You will be told to what extent amyloid plaques and fibrillary tangles were found. This will give you closure that you were in fact dealing with Alzheimer's disease. Or you may be told that your loved one suffered from one of the other forms of dementia described. Brain tissue can then be used in research to find a solution to these most vexing and puzzling diseases. If you follow this course, you and your loved one will have contributed to what is our highest goal for the future: a world without Alzheimer's disease.

What Causes Death in Alzheimer's Patients?

The cause of death of an Alzheimer's patient can vary widely, but generally he or she will die either from Alzheimer's disease itself or from any variety of other causes. Alzheimer's disease can cause death directly by one of several mechanisms: a common cause is bronchopneumonia, as impairment of reflexes allows secretions to accumulate in the bronchial tree; or aspiration pneumonia, as the swallowing mechanism becomes impaired in the late stages. A drop in blood pressure, as the automatic mechanisms for maintaining normal blood pressure become impaired, can also cause death. Non-Alzheimer's-related causes, too, can occur at any stage of the disease—fatal accidents, strokes, cancer, heart attacks, or infections, for instance, can happen to Alzheimer's patients just as if they can to any one of us. Accordingly, you should not be too surprised if the diagnosis of Alzheimer's disease does not appear on your loved one's death certificate.

Gather Those Who Are Dear to You

This is the time to gather around you those who are dearest to you. They will share in your grief and remember with you the one you have lost. Memories of the one you loved will remain forever, even though his or her own memories disappeared tragically before their time. And these loved ones will help you remember that no one else could have done what you have done. All those who understand your efforts will be grateful to you forever.

Chapter Summary

1. Along with grief, you may also experience a sense of relief when your loved one dies. There is no need to have feelings of guilt over that sense of relief.

2. This is the last chance to decide whether to have a brain autopsy performed on your loved one.

3. Now is the time to gather around you those who are dear to you. All those who understand what you have accomplished will be forever grateful to you.

Chapter 20

Recovery from Caregiving

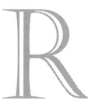ELATIVELY little attention has been paid in other books on Alzheimer's disease and dementia to the period in caregivers' lives that begins after the death of their patients. Yet I think this one of the most important in the story of caregiving. As Helen in the Postscript says: "There *is* life after Alzheimer's." Some caregivers initially feel that they will never fully recover from the experience of caregiving. With persistent effort, however, I believe that you can and must fully recover, for at least one important reason: you are now in a much better position to take advantage of all the opportunities that life still has waiting for you.

Being a Caregiver Will Have Changed You

When you really "wake up" from caregiving, you will find that you are now a changed person in a number of ways:

- You have learned that you can adapt to ever-changing circumstances
- You have learned that you can be far more creative than you had ever imagined
- You have learned just how strong and re-sourceful you are
- You have learned how to give unconditional love over an extended period of time

Of course the exact nature of these changes will vary widely from person to person, but in general these wonderful qualities are either learned or enhanced as part of the caregiving experience.

You will also discover that you have lived through a lengthy period of severe stress, and that too has left its mark on you. You will discover leftover scars and wounds that need healing, and so may from time to time be overcome by strong emotions such as severe sadness, guilt, or anger. In some ways these experiences resemble flashbacks such as those experienced in post-traumatic stress disorders. If this happens to you, be assured that you are not the only one. Many caregivers have told me that they were very surprised when they first experienced these feelings, and they didn't quite know what to make of them. What it means is the long period of stress, of isolation, or limiting your personal life to caregiving has done some damage. And that you will now need to take the initiative to help yourself achieve a full recovery from caregiving.

Esther, whom I quoted earlier, continued to blog about her caregiver experience after her patient's death, and a number of these blogs were published in a column for her hometown paper, the *Seattle Post and Intelligencer,* under the title *Witnessing Alzheimer's: A Caregiver's View.* Here is one such column that I think is particularly tellingly observed and articulately presented:

I can get mad at him again

I don't have to go to the nursing home anymore. I don't even have to think about going. Not today, not tomorrow. Not next week. And I can get mad at him again. Isn't that an odd thing to be thinking? I didn't get mad at him the whole time he was in the nursing home, three years and ten months. Not once, a contrast—you can be sure—from before he became ill.

I can't understand how life can go on as usual. Buses run, shoppers shop, the grocery store on the corner still stands. Starbucks hasn't gone out of business. Facebook flourishes. Yet Abe is in the ground. He's wrapped in a shroud. . . . He's gone. He flickered on earth for a while, and then he left.

While I'm still at his bedside, asking him for one more breath, I have him back with me as he used to be; and he is saying to all who knew and loved him: "Thank you, you helped me through." To me he's saying, as . . . I was watching the shovels of dirt hit his coffin: "You did it, Babe. You got me buried, and I'm proud."

Now I have to remember how I used to be before he got sick. The sound of my voice is unfamiliar. The name of the day. Time is different. I didn't realize there were so many hours to use as I wish. My life is trying to reach me, before I sleep. I think it will.

What Does It Take to Recover from Caregiving?

Actually, a lot. You will want to undertake a whole set of coordinated activities in order to become "whole" again. Of course, time is a powerful healer, but time alone will not be enough. First, you will want to rebuild your social network. This will involve telling friends and acquaintances that you are "back": you will want to become socially more active, attend parties, or perhaps give a party to demonstrate that you are back. And you will start to accept invitations to parties again.

You will also want to resume regular vigorous exercise, preferably with others, and to use optimal nutrition to support your recovery. This will mean including lots of fruits and vegetables in your diet, and minimizing anything containing refined sugar or refined flour. You will also need to assure that you have an adequate intake of healthy fats, lean protein, and ample vitamins.

You will be able to resume a much more regular sleep pattern, so aim for a healthy seven to eight hours of sleep, going to bed and arising at the same time each day. And practice whatever stress-reducing strategies that work for you, whether this means meditation, yoga or tai chi, or just regular times for deep breathing. Of course spending time with trusted friends whenever new stresses occur will also help.

You now have the freedom to seek out pleasurable activities on a regular basis and even indulgences of which you have probably long been deprived. Go for it!

And along the way, don't forget to offer and receive love from friends and relatives. Household pets can also provide and accept unconditional love. Just being next to and petting an animal we love is a great stress reducer and a way to feel good about ourselves.

You can also reconnect with your spiritual life, which may have suffered during your long period of caregiving. This may include religious or nonreligious forms of spirituality, as well as regular experiences in nature. I have long been a believer in the creative and curative benefits of communing with nature.

For some individuals supportive counseling with a mental health professional may also be needed for a full recovery. You should not hesitate to access such help if you experience depression or frequent attacks of anxiety.

Write Your Future

As you imagine your new life unfolding, document your ideas by writing them down. It is well known that a written plan is far more likely to be accomplished than is a general idea. Make your plan as detailed as you can envision it. Then picture it in your mind, not only seeing what you are planning to achieve, but also visualizing how it would feel to execute what you have sketched out. Finally, start to implement it, one step at a time. Make adjustments in your plans if needed, and overcome obstacles to your plan through persistence and endurance.

As part of this healing process, you may want to establish a whole new set of goals for the remaining part of your life. What this may include will depend at what stage in life you are when your caregiving is over. If you have been a caregiver for a spouse of a similar age to yours, the time remaining might only be somewhere between five and fifteen years. If you have been caring for a parent, you may be only in your fifties or sixties, and you will have a whole generation of life left to live, anywhere from ten to thirty-five years. So what I recommend is that you first start by jotting down things that you might still wish to accomplish or to experience; then begin to prioritize them; then begin to discuss them with friends, confidantes or counselors, or members of your caregiver group. This will be a most important undertaking for you. What I am recommending is that you literally write your future.

How Long Does It Take to Recover?

Six months? A year? The rest of your life? Well, somewhere in between, depending on how actively you work on getting back on your feet emotionally and physically. Esther, the caregiver whom I have quoted elsewhere in this book, continues to write poems to and about her husband. Her latest book jacket shows her with a confident, serene smile. Esther has given me permission to quote a sequence of her poems here. Esther, I want you to feel *whole* again!

With permission, then, I quote here from Esther Altshul Helfgott's book *Listening to Mozart: Poems of Alzheimer's* (Yakima, WA: Cave Moon Press, 2014):

> I wish I could find you
> in my dreams—
> you must be busy
> —what are you doing
> that's so important
>
> it's 10 o'clock
> and I'm still in bed
> thinking of you
> not here

today—
again

I wonder
which galaxy
you're in
now—
are we still
under the same
moon

a leaf falls
I watch
you pick it up
you
disappear

Continue to Attend Your Caregiver Support Group

A number of caregivers I know have continued to attend their support groups. There they not only continue to receive the love and affection of other group members, but also share that they themselves are now "recovering," and will soon be ready to resume a new and a full life that might include anything. And what might that "anything" be for you? Perhaps you will want to consider some or all of these possibilities:

Help other caregivers or fundraise for Alzheimer's research. You might apply the knowledge you have gained to help other people struggling with caregiving tasks. Certainly there is a great need for this, and you would feel rewarded for teaching others what you have learned during your long career as a caregiver. Or you might become a fundraiser for Alzheimer's disease research, since you know so well that further progress in this area is desperately needed.

Write a book about your caregiving experience. If you decided to write a book about your caregiver experience, you would have much to share, and many would be grateful for what they could learn from your journey. An interesting variation on this theme might be for you to write a book about the person for whom you provided care. Now there is an idea!

Try an entirely new direction. You may wish instead to turn completely away from having any further dealings with this disease, and pursue all those activities that had to be put on the back burner during your caregiving career. This might include reconnecting with other family members or friends whom you may have had to neglect while caregiving, or to pursue other creative or spiritual activities. A long and a long-delayed vacation would certainly be something you deserve, and which you can now enjoy.

You Are a Modern Day Hero. Thank You!

Whatever activities you may wish to undertake, you will be able to do so with greater skills and confidence than you ever had before. You have grown, you have matured, and you have extended your capabilities to where there is nothing that you cannot do. Nothing could be more difficult than what you have been through. I personally believe that you as a caregiver of someone with Alzheimer's disease have truly been a modern hero or heroine. Congratulations! Well done! You have every reason to be truly proud of yourself. The power of your shining example will be there for others to follow. On behalf of all the patients who can no longer say it themselves: thank you, thank you, thank you.

CHAPTER SUMMARY

1. Little has been written about recovery from caregiving, but it's an essential part of every caregiver's life story.

2. Recovery from caregiving is a process that takes care and determination to complete. Make sure to take good care of yourself and to make a written plan of what you want your future to look like.

3. Continue to attend your caregiver support group as you work out the next steps in this new life stage, and reach out to other family and friends as you reconnect to those who love you and can support you.

Postscript

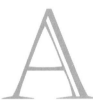FTER finishing a first draft of the manuscript for this book, I felt the need to reconnect with some of the most successful caregivers I had come to know over a period of some thirty years. After some reflection on what I, and by extension you, could still learn from them, I called together a group of seven experienced caregivers, two men and five women, for a Sunday afternoon get-together to reflect on their caregiver experiences.

The individuals I gathered were basically strangers, or at best, acquaintances. Yes, they all had in common their caregiver experience and they knew why they had gathered. But when they met, something special happened. There was instant rapport of a kind that no one seemed to have expected. They opened up and trusted people they barely knew with some very raw emotions and memories that they had never shared with anyone. It was a deeply surprising and very moving experience. We all felt very close to one another, and I believe we all felt exceedingly privileged to be with one another on that afternoon.

Each member of the group had read the manuscript sometime during the preceding week, and each in turn expressed the feeling that they wished such a book had been available to them when they had begun their caregiving experience. Nearly everyone that afternoon said they wanted to make copies of the book available to their friends who were just now facing a similar challenge.

I asked each of them to respond to five questions. Each gave very thoughtful, widely differing responses to these questions that I think you will find enlightening. I first tried to summarize their responses, but came to feel that that I could not do full justice to their wisdom and their creativity. Accordingly, I am going to let all of them speak for themselves. Each member gave permission to have his or her words included in this section. So here are the five questions, and the responses of each of my seven caregiver friends.

What Was the Hardest Thing about Your Caregiving Experience?

Helen: "That was almost thirty years ago. Nobody had ever heard of Alzheimer's disease. It was hard because you feel so isolated. It really separates your friends from your acquaintances. It was exhausting, it was draining. Even when you are out with friends, it sits on your shoulder. And, of course, your heart is broken."

John: "Sending my wife to a facility, even though it was the best thing for both of us."

Pat G.: "The only thing that was available then was a nursing home. And they were really still very understaffed then. The other thing that was hard for me was to see my Mom let the nurses do things for her that she wouldn't let me do."

Ed: "Seeing the gradual decline of my mother-in-law over a number of years."

Pat B.: "The loneliness. The isolation that I felt and that he felt, too. I wondered if people felt the disease was contagious. They wouldn't come near him, they wouldn't touch him. Only one person, a close friend, came to greet us and touch him. Your friends stop talking to you. They stay away."

Shirley: "Not having my Mom to talk to any more. And the role change when I was suddenly the parent and she the child."

Dolly: "Putting my Mom in the Assisted Living Unit. It was terrible to see her distress and confusion. That really got to me, and it still does." (At this point, she broke into tears.)

What Was the Most Rewarding Part of Your Caregiver Experience?

Helen: "Was there anything rewarding? It was very hard. I guess I was glad that I finally got some help. I finally understood what to expect next. That was a blessing. I felt compelled to do this since he had taken such wonderful care of me and the children for so many years."

John: "I didn't find it very rewarding. But I felt rewarded by being able to help others in the support group based on what I had learned."

Pat G.: "It taught me about Alzheimer's disease. It was also very rewarding that my Mom knew me until she died. I always felt she knew me, even when she thought I was her mother."

Ed: "It prompted me to assist one of the first caregiver support groups in the area to become an Alzheimer's Association Chapter, which I then ran for six years."

Pat B.: "During the time it didn't seem very rewarding. But looking back, it was a real education. I learned humility. I learned to arrange life so that it suited both of us, not just me alone. I kept taking him to our place of business, and I kept him so well dressed and groomed that many people didn't even know he was ill."

Shirley: "Yes, there were many rewards, and I made the commitment to it, even though I had to retire twelve years early from my job. I loved finding little things to do with her, like reciting nursery rhymes that she remembered or singing songs together. 'You Are My Sunshine' was her favorite, and we sang it everywhere, in the doctor's office, or in the car, and I don't care that people stared at us."

Dolly: "The little things. That I could still spend quality time with my Mom. Yes, I was glad that I was available to help. I knew she had always loved puzzles. So I would find or invent simple puzzles that she could still do, and we would do them together."

What Was the Best Advice Anyone Gave You about Your Caregiver Tasks?

Helen: "You can't argue with them."

John: "The doctor was worried about my health condition. So he told me to take her to a facility. What was surprising was that she settled in fairly well, without a lot of distress on her part. She accepted it."

Pat G.: "Bringing familiar things to her room at the facility. I was told to get help, to get out of the 'I can do it alone' mode. And to get help when the patient can still form a relationship with other helpers."

Ed: "There will be conflict, and misbehavior. But it will not be willful on the part of the patient. It is the disease. Don't do battle with the person; you may just have to walk away for a bit."

Pat B.: "Take care of yourself! The patient could outlive you if you died or were to fall apart."

Shirley: "Not a lot of advice was available. I had to go through a lot of trial and error. You need so much *patience!* And what works today will not necessarily work tomorrow. You have to keep adapting. When my Mom would not take a bath, I said, 'We are going to make you queen for a day.' Her name was Elizabeth, and I would call her Queen Elizabeth, and we would go to the spa in our own bathroom, and she would have her hair done and look really beautiful. That way she took a bath with happiness and pleasure."

Dolly: "Go to a caregiver conference! It really helped. I learned so much in one day. I also learned about going to 'post-graduation' caregiver support groups."

What Advice Would You Give Someone Just Starting Out on the Caregiver Experience?

Helen: "Find a support group, and get help early. If there is a university in your community, see what it has to offer."

John: "You've got to belong to a caregiver group. You might even join more than one, because they have different things to offer. When you can't take care of the person any longer, it is not a reflection on you."

Pat G.: "Get an elder-law attorney early while you both can still participate."

Ed: "Begin the organization of family resources as soon as the diagnosis has been made. Identify necessary and qualified medical and legal support services. Develop and implement a checklist to follow. Include other family members from the beginning."

Pat B.: "For our fiftieth anniversary we had a big celebration. A lot of people came and he just sat there. That evening he didn't remember a thing. But it is still important to do those kinds of things for the person. It was also important to me and to my daughter."

Dolly: "Pass on the advice that you get. Learn extreme patience. Remember you are not dealing with your Mom or Dad, but with a new person who has the illness."

What Other Topics Should Be Included in a Book on Caregiving in Alzheimer's Disease?

Helen: "There *is* life after Alzheimer's!"

John: "That there are other forms of dementia, such as vascular dementia, Lewy body disease, and normal pressure hydrocephalus."

Pat G.: "The need for long-distance caregiving."

Ed G.: "Right at the beginning, when the diagnosis is first made, there is the need for power of attorney and for a healthcare surrogate. Make sure that the larger family understands what is needed and why it is needed."

Pat B.: "Make this book available to any new caregiver, even those caring for people with other diseases. They can learn from the Alzheimer's caregiver experience."

Shirley: "Tell people where they can find information. Also, to know about adult protective services for people who don't have a caregiver."

Dolly: "This book needs to go to doctors as well as caregivers, and to relatives and friends, so that they understand what the caregiver is going through."

Wow! There was a whole lot of wisdom, and a huge amount of emotion in that room that Sunday afternoon. There was not a dry eye in the house. I hope that I have done justice to all the participants. But my experience with them that day confirms what I have suspected all along: when you want to fully understand what you have been going through while caring for your loved one with Alzheimer's disease, connect with a support group. Even after your experience is over, you can call a group of your former support group members and share your remembrances. Just be sure to have plenty of tissues on hand.

Appendix:
Resources for Caregivers and Families

In this section I am going to discuss a number of resources that have helped caregivers like you at various stages of their loved one's disease, and at different times during their caregiving experience. You might browse through this section and read about those resources that strike you as relevant, keeping in mind that some may be more useful at some point later on in your caregiving.

Adult Protective Services

People with Alzheimer's disease who are living alone or who don't have any family member or close friend who could provide care should be referred to social service agencies. If you learn of such a person who is living alone without support, be sure to let the police or elder care charity in that person's neighborhood know. The patient can then be referred or admitted to special assisted-living facilities where many of the services that would be offered by a family caregiver can be provided by a professional trained caregiver.

Alzheimer's Association

The Alzheimer's Association is the largest nationwide advocacy organization in support of individuals affected by Alzheimer's disease. It provides a description of the disease as well as information about diagnostic and treatment services, caregiver support services, and other issues of significance. It has local chapters in many communities throughout the United States. The association also has a significant lobbying arm that seeks to influence federal legislation related to Alzheimer's disease research and services. To contact the association, call its twenty-four-hour helpline at 800-272-3900, or use your internet browser to visit www.alz.org.

Area Agencies on Aging

Area Agencies on Aging are federally funded community organizations designed to assist elderly persons in finding health, social, respite, and other services. They can also help you find volunteer opportunities, meal service sites, and senior centers as well as respite care programs. Every sizeable community has one or is served by one. They can be found in your local phone books under a listing of federal government agencies, or through the national Eldercare Locator (800-677-1116 or www.eldercare.gov).

Assisted Living Facilities

Assisted living facilities, or ALFs, are residential facilities that provide basic food and shelter for people who are no longer able to provide these for themselves. Care in ALFs is not covered by Medicare or Medicaid, but it is specifically covered by some long-term care insurance policies. Some ALFs provide assistance only with basic self-care while others may additionally provide medication administration and medical monitoring, such as blood pressure measurements or blood sugar testing.

There are generalized assisted living facilities as well as specialized ALFs that focus solely on memory-impaired patients. If such specialized facilities are available, these should be chosen over general ALFs.

Caregiver Seminars

At the University of South Florida we began to conduct caregiver training seminars for individuals engaged at all levels of caregiving for an Alzheimer's patient. These are day-long learning sessions in which all aspects of Alzheimer's disease and all aspects of caregiving are discussed by a series of experts on medical, social, legal, and financial aspects of caregiving. Caregivers are encouraged to ask questions and present problems to these experts for solutions. These caregiver seminars have been described as "lifesavers" by many participants. If your community does not yet offer such training sessions, discuss this possibility with the medical or social service staff of the memory clinic you are attending, and encourage them to "go and do likewise."

Eldercare Locator

The Eldercare Locator is a public service provided by the Administration on Aging of the U.S. government. It provides a listing of all Area Agencies on Aging as well as all State Units on Aging. Through your local Area Agency on Aging you can find access to community health care, nutrition, home care, and caregiver services. To get started, contact the Eldercare Locator at 800-677-1116 or www.eldercare.gov.

Long-Distance Caregiving

Many caregivers do not reside close to their patient's home or care facility. In this situation, I recommend that a local geriatric care manager be employed who can coordinate doctor visits, medication-taking, daycare or respite care, or eventual admission to a care facility. Just as the patient cannot report accurately on his or her memory problems or problems in living, neither will you be able to assess the problems long distance. Your local Alzheimer's Association chapter or Area Agency on Aging may be able to put you in touch with a geriatric care manager. An initial personal visit to where the patient lives is also recommended, with return visits as often as is feasible.

Long-Term Care Insurance

Insurance can provide for the cost of receiving long-term care for a chronic illness that you or your spouse may develop. Depending on the specific terms of your long-term care insurance policy, this can include the cost of a nursing home, an assisted living facility, or medical care that you receive in your home. The reason for insuring against long-term care costs is that these costs can be very high indeed, and may continue over months or even years. The cost of nursing home care may range anywhere from $60,000 to $120,000 a year, depending on where in the country this cost is incurred, with the highest costs being experienced in the Northeast and California, and the lowest costs being charged in the Southern states. Thus over a period of several years, the cost of nursing home care can completely wipe out a considerable fortune.

The cost of long-term care insurance can be very reasonable and affordable if it is purchased for an individual who is still generally healthy. By contrast, the cost of such insurance for someone who already has a condition that is likely to result in long-term care, such as diabetes with complications or Alzheimer's disease, is almost always prohibitively expensive and often is not much less than the cost of paying for such care out of pocket. Moreover, once the disease has been diagnosed in an individual, it is unlikely that such a person will be granted this type of insurance. So it would be wise to acquire it when the person to be covered is still free of any serious chronic disease.

The practical lesson to be learned from this discussion is that while it may be too late to acquire long-term care insurance for your loved one affected with Alzheimer's disease, it may be just the right time to purchase such insurance for yourself while you are still in good health and while rates are still very reasonable for you.

Acknowledgments

It gives me great pleasure to acknowledge with profound gratitude a number of individuals who have made the development of this book possible and who share a great deal of the credit for helping it reach caregivers like you.

Jean Thomson Black, senior executive editor at Yale University Press, provided the critical "Yes" by first inviting a detailed proposal for the book and subsequently extending a publishing offer to me. The editor who had accepted my earlier book on health and wellness, *Winning Strategies for Successful Aging,* she took a considerable leap of faith by agreeing to publish a previously self-published book while suggesting major expansions and additions to the original work.

Dr. Julie Silver, at the Harvard School of Medicine

Writer's Workshop, encouraged and enabled me to proceed to completion of the book, and introduced me to Jean Thomson Black. She instilled confidence and courage to proceed along the lines I had originally sketched out, while encouraging me to reach as many readers as possible with the advice and support that my manuscript contained.

Lisa Tener, a writing coach from Rhode Island participating as faculty member in Julie Silver's writing workshop, provided inspiration and practical know-how for moving from the idea stage to a finished manuscript. I am extremely grateful to her for believing in my message and allowing me to amplify my voice to the point where it can do the most good.

Gia Metcalf, my dear friend and neighbor, provided computer and formatting skills that I completely lacked. Thank you, Gia, for helping in such a facile and elegant way, and for being willing to come back time and again to get me unstuck, all while expressing confidence that the project was very much worthwhile.

Dolly Williams, a former caregiver, great friend, editor, and powerful advocate for caregivers, served as my "grammar police" and came up with many suggestions for additional content not previously covered—and did so in a manner that almost made it seem as if the ideas had come from me. I owe her a huge debt of gratitude.

John Luce, also a former caregiver and a friend, provided a husband's perspective on caregiving as he went from first admitting his wife had a problem, to acquiring a definitive diagnosis, to caregiving over many years both at home and in an assisted living facility, to experiencing her death, and all the way toward achieving a full recovery from the caregiver experience. John was amazingly eager to share what he had learned with other caregivers. He not only writes about caregiving but also has conducted caregiver groups as well as caregiver classes. He did this to such an extent and with such devotion in relation to my project that he functioned as a virtual co-author of the book. Thank you, thank you, John.

Esther Altshul Helfgott, caregiver of her pathologist husband for almost ten years, storyteller, and poet, allowed me to include two of her stories and a sequence of her poems in this volume. She is a remarkably keen observer and a very articulate writer. She helped me especially to flesh out my thoughts on recovery from caregiving.

Natasha Pfeiffer, my beloved wife of fifty years (together we have been married for a hundred years!) read every word I wrote innumerable times, told me in the kindest way possible where I was not quite clear, where my sentences were awkward (we called it "finding auks") and where my language was still too technical to be easily understood. She also provided enormous encouragement that allowed me to proceed when I had seemingly reached a dead end. My gratitude to her is simply endless.

Julie Carlson, a manuscript editor for Yale University Press, brought improved organization and greater clarity to my presentation while totally honoring my authorial intent. She also provided more felicitous language where needed to make the book "sing."

Helen Gibbons, Pat Geasa and Ed Geasa, Pat Bunch, and Shirley Temple rounded out the "gang of seven" who met with me after reading the manuscript and contributed their wisdom and creativity to the Postscript.

Finally, I am grateful to all the caregivers it has been my privilege to know and from whom I have learned so much. It is your experience and advice that have shaped my message, a message that I am now happy to pass on to all the caregivers in all the world ("tout le monde"). Thank you!

Index

INDEX

amyloid, 120
amyloid beta 42 peptide, 84,
    87–88
amyloid PET scanning, 84–85
amyloid plaques, 84, 87
anger: in caregivers, 21–22, 23,
    227; in patients, 22, 23
anhedonia, 178–179
anti-anxiety medications, 107,
    111
antibiotics, 120
antidepressants, 96, 107, 119,
    178–179, 180
antipsychotic medications, 75,
    107
anxiety, 74, 111, 156, 165, 231
apathy, 96, 178–179
ApoE gene, 86–87, 121
Area Agencies on Aging, 33,
    148, 249, 251
Aricept, 55, 82, 92–93, 105, 119,
    183
arrhythmia, 25, 102
arthritis, 73
aspiration pneumonia, 224
aspirin, 120
assisted living facilities, 24,
    187, 191, 210, 211, 216, 248,
    249–250, 252
athletics, 108, 110
atrophy, of brain, 64, 84
attention deficit/hyperactivity
    disorder (ADHD), 178
autopsy, 80, 85, 156–157, 173,
    223–224, 225
Axona, 94

bank accounts, 129
bathing, 162
bathroom habits, 144–145, 157,
    161, 181–182, 189, 191

battlefield injuries, 108
behavioral problems, 89, 141;
    disruptive, 12, 93, 96; in
    early stages, 145–146;
    exercising to improve, 97;
    in late stages, 174, 189;
    management of, 95–96, 107,
    142, 154; medications to
    improve, 98; in middle
    stages, 157, 165–168; types
    of, 65
benign forgetfulness, 51–53, 56
blood count, 83
blood pressure, 224, 250
blood sugar, 83, 250
blood tests, 84, 87–88
boxing, 108
brain donation, 44–45,
    156–157, 173, 223–224, 225
brainstem, 103
brain trauma, 57, 58, 67, 89
brain tumors, 172
broken bones, 74, 77, 181
bronchopneumonia, 224
"bucket lists," 134
burnout, 13, 208, 214

calorie counts, 164
Cameron, David, 122
cancer, 164, 188, 224
cardiologists, 102
caregivers, caregiving: adult
    children as, 22–23, 27;
    anger in, 21–22, 23, 227;
    assistants recruited for,
    213–214; buddy system in,
    35, 38; burnout and, 13,
    208, 214; child rearing vs.,
    32; choosing, 15–16; classes
    for, 13; clinical detachment
    in, 141–142; commitment

About the Author

Dr. Eric Pfeiffer is a nationally and internationally recognized authority on health and aging. He is the founding director of the Suncoast Alzheimer's and Gerontology Center at the University of South Florida College of Medicine, and the author of several major textbooks on health and aging, including *Behavior and Adaptation in Late Life* and *Mental Illness in Late Life*, both published by Little, Brown. He is now retired from medical practice and devotes his time to writing and speaking to lay and professional audiences about successful aging and about caregiving in Alzheimer's disease.

In 1977 Dr. Pfeiffer was awarded the Allen Gold Medal for outstanding achievement in the area of Geriatric Psychiatry by the American Geriatric Society. In 1985 Dr. Pfeiffer was honored for his work in the area of

Alzheimer's disease through the establishment of the Eric Pfeiffer Chair in Alzheimer's Disease Research at the University of South Florida. Most recently, Dr. Pfeiffer has been nominated for the Senior Living Media Award of the Florida Council on Aging, largely on the basis of his two most recent books, *Winning Strategies for Successful Aging* published by Yale University Press (2013) and *The Art of Caregiving in Alzheimer's Disease* published by Amazon (2012).

Dr. Pfeiffer has conducted numerous studies on new medications for use with Alzheimer's patients and individuals with minor cognitive impairment. These studies include work with the cholinesterase inhibitors Aricept, Exelon, and Razadyne, as well as with Namenda. His work has been published widely in many scientific journals on topics related to health, mental health, and aging. He has also lectured at many universities, colleges, and professional organizations.

Dr. Pfeiffer is also a published poet. His first book of poetry, *Take with Me Now That Enormous Step,* was winner of the Charioteer Poetry Award. His second book of poems, entitled *Under One Roof,* has just been published. Some of his poems have appeared in *Journal of the American Medical Association (JAMA)* and in *The Pharos.*

ABOUT THE AUTHOR

You can learn more about Dr. Pfeiffer's scheduled public presentations and appearances, as well as other activities, by visiting his website, www.DoctorEricKnows .com. On the website you will see a blog about caregiving, a sample of his recent poems, his contact information, and other resources for caregivers. Dr. Pfeiffer welcomes comments from his readers.